The Food Freedom Formula
Intuitive Eating for Every Body

By Lana Nelson

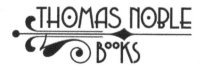

Copyright © 2018 Lana Nelson. All rights reserved. No portion of this book may be reproduced mechanically, electronically, or by any other means, including photocopying, without written permission from the author. It is illegal to copy this book, post it to a website, or distribute it by any other means without permission from the author.

Author Contact: TheFoodCodes.com

Thomas Noble Books

Wilmington, DE

www.thomasnoblebooks.com

Library of Congress Control Number: 2018955080

ISBN: 978-1-945586-12-5

First Printing: 2018

Editing by Gwen Hoffnagle

Cover Design by Sarah Barrie of Cyanotype.ca

This publication is designed to provide accurate and authoritative information regarding the subject matter covered. It is sold with the understanding that the author is not engaged in rendering professional services. If legal, accounting, medical, psychological, or any other expert assistance is required, the services of a competent professional person should be sought. Client names have been changed to protect identities.

DEDICATION

To Dr. Bruce A. Nelson, D.C., my gifted husband, who introduced me to the miracles of natural healing. He healed my body from ten long years of constant pain and healed my heart and my children with his love. He has the kindest heart I know and has created great fun and adventure since the day he proposed to me, dressed in a gorilla suit.

To The Brady Bunch Times Two. That's what the newspaper headlines called us when Bruce adopted my six children: Jennifer, Natalie, Will, Matt, Adam, and Jonathan, and we combined his six kids: Rachel, Matt, Courtney, David, Ashley, and Whitney, to make a clan of *our* twelve children. The love and friendship we have astounds people.

To the spouses of my children. Thank you for being such amazing people and parenting the most brilliant grandchildren on the planet!

I love you all.

Table of Contents

The Food Codes 7
    Chapter 1:   Can You Make Food Your Friend 9
    Chapter 2:   Why Diets Don't Work 19
    Chapter 3:   Understanding Food's Role 25
    Chapter 4:   The Impact of Emotions on Your Weight,
                    Food, and How You Eat It 43
    Chapter 5:   Muscle-Testing 55

The Food Codes System 81
    Chapter 6:   Unlocking Your Food Codes 83
    Chapter 7:   Living Well with Your Food Codes Plan 97
    Chapter 8:   Improving the Way Your Body Uses Food 109
    Chapter 9:   Feeling Great All the Time 129
    Chapter 10: Intentional Eating – The Art of Enjoying
                    Your Food and Your Life 145

Cooking and Recipes 159
    Chapter 11: Reconnecting with Food 161
    Chapter 12: Getting Ready to Cook 171
    Chapter 13: Recipes 185
    Chapter 14: Cooking with the Food Codes 239

    Appendix 1: Measurement Conversion Chart 265
    Appendix 2: Measurement Conversions for Pans
                    and Dishes 267
    Appendix 3: Oven Temperature Conversions 269

    About the Author 271
    Acknowledgments 273
    Get More from Lana 275

The Food Codes

CHAPTER 1
Can You Make Food Your Friend?

First we eat, then we do everything else.
— M. F. K. Fisher

Consider all the close relationships you've had in life. Can you identify your very first relationship? It was with food!

After you were conceived, the nutrition you received inside your mother was key to your development. You were sheltered in a womb that gave you oxygen, nutrition, and water. In fact, food was so important to your growing body that if your mother did not consume enough calcium to support you, her body provided it from her teeth and bones. As soon as you were born you were fed, either from your mother's body or from a bottle of formula. A baby who is not fed will not live.

Food has been a part of your life from the very beginning, even before you had conscious memories. It has sustained you, comforted you, entertained you, and, if you are like most people in Western countries, has also been a source of shame and conflict.

We are rarely happy about our relationship with food. We eat too much or starve ourselves in an effort to match society's ideas of what is beautiful and healthy. We try diets that don't work for us, read books and articles about what we should and should not eat, and mindlessly eat chips or chocolate when we are stressed.

Most of us are confused and frustrated about food. Experts tell us what foods to eat, but the recommendations change all the time. A friend goes on a diet and gets into her skinny jeans, but you gain weight following the same diet.

We also feel guilty about food. We eat fast food in our cars, keep a stash of emergency snacks for bad days at work, and sometimes fail to give our bodies the nutrition they need. Our emotions swing between feeling motivated and ready to get our eating under control and giving up completely and standing in the kitchen eating ice cream from the carton.

Does this sound like the relationship you'd have with a true friend?

Pause for a long moment to think about what gives you joy and comfort. Do your thoughts distill down to simple things like a heart-to-heart hug, settling into a comfy chair with a good book and a warm mug of tea, or maybe a lovely meal with someone you love while you reminisce over happy times together? Ah yes, the creature comforts of good food, friendly relationships, and comfortable accommodations – those simple joys – truly make life sweet and easy and aren't many of your memories of joyous times intertwined with your good friend, food?

The Food Codes is about getting to know food at a deeper and more intimate level. It's about considering food as a whole, living, energy being. Food has been our friend from the time of our very conception, yet most of us barely know her. We have taken her and her presence for granted more than anything else we have ever been given. We have used and abused her. She is the most misunderstood soul on this planet.

We dig deeply into understanding our inner selves and our relationships with others. We turn each other inside out to find more connectedness. However, there is one relationship left wanting, and that is our relationship with food.

Many of us feel a push/pull relationship with food. We strive to control our food intake and often feel helpless about what we eat. We want to control our appetites and eating because we secretly feel out of control and helpless. Food is seen as a temptation, a comfort, a hassle, and a constant balancing act. How many times have you said, "I know this is bad for me, but I'm going to eat it, anyway"? It can almost feel like you are committing adultery or a deadly sin when you eat something you crave that you believe is bad for you.

Think about how much energy you spend worrying about what you eat. Wouldn't it be wonderful to let go of that burden?

In *The Food Codes* you'll discover that you can become friends with food and enjoy a healthy, nourishing, empowering relationship. When you follow the Food Codes and make food your friend, you'll know its heart. You'll become comfortable with food because you'll know exactly how to determine what foods will give you optimal health each day. Any guilt you feel about food will disappear. You'll learn to listen to what your body needs, whether it's fresh broccoli or a piece of chocolate cake. When you are following your Food Codes plan, all the drama and confusion regarding food fades away.

Your body has a miraculous way of showing you precisely what it needs for optimal health and wellness. Your body and your inner knower – your intuition – already understand the Food Codes. The solutions to your challenges with food are already inside you! You only need to learn some simple tools to access them.

Once you renew your friendship with food and learn simple ways to access your unique Food Codes, you'll have vitality and wellness and be able to easily maintain your ideal weight. This might sound too good to be true, yet it is true. Your relationship with food can be positive and simple.

Philosopher and naturalist Henry David Thoreau wrote:

> *I do believe in simplicity. When the mathematician would solve a difficult problem, he first frees the equation of all encumbrances and reduces it to its simplest terms. So simplify the problem of life, distinguish the necessary and the real. Probe the earth to see where your main roots run.*

Finding the best foods for yourself and those you love does not have to be a complex issue anymore. You don't have to be a food research scientist to know what is good for you to eat. You don't have to guess or ask others for their opinions or advice. *The Food Codes* gives you the simplest way on the planet to know what foods are good for you. This book is intended to be an easy learning guide. Your body works in complex ways, but you'll read about them in very simple terms.

Albert Einstein said, "If you can't explain it to a six year old, you don't understand it yourself." There are children as young as five who are able to use the methods you will read about in *The Food Codes*. Yet simple does not mean ineffective. There are doctors who use the Food Codes method in their professional practices. I've used it for twenty years with many patients and clients, testing and revising it over time until I am confident it works with all kinds of people. It does!

My client Marty suffered from low energy, breathing problems, heart palpitations, bulging veins, and painful throbbing all over her body. She'd seen numerous doctors who could not find a long-lasting cure. After I taught her the Food Codes method, she found that some of the foods she'd been told to strictly avoid were exactly what she needed to eat to heal. She followed her Food Codes for one month just to see what would happen. After a month she had more energy, her heart palpitations had disappeared, and her pain was gone. By listening to what her body needed instead of what other people told her, she was able to heal.

Pain, Miracles, and Food

In 1993 I was in a terrible car accident. There was an accident in front of me that caused me to stop, and then a semi-truck slammed into the back of my car. The collision impacted my head and neck. Over the next ten years I had severe migraines, pain in my jaw and face and shooting pain all over my body. Physical therapy and evaluations by occupational retraining experts determined that there was no job I could be retrained for, due to the constant daily pain I experienced.

I was sent to neurologists for the throbbing headaches and seizure-like spells that kept occurring. Muscle relaxers and pain pills were prescribed. I was naïve because I had never taken much medication in my life. I thought the drugs would cure the pain. Wrong! The pain-killers and muscle-relaxers made me incoherent and did not release me from the pain.

Then I started having severe pains in my abdomen that sent me to the emergency room, where I received the diagnosis of diverticulitis, a swelling in the bowel. My bowel continued to flare up, causing cramps that doubled me over and lasted for days. I was a single mom with six little children, so I really struggled while fighting all the problems in my body and trying to take care of my family.

As you can imagine, I was ready to try anything that would help, including some pretty funny things like "slant board therapy" – sleeping with my feet elevated above my head on my ironing board, which was propped up at a slant at the foot of my bed. My two little boys walked barefoot on my back when I researched Oriental massage techniques. (Don't try this! You might end up with two kids trying to play King of the Mountain on your back, which always resulted in someone crashing down hard on the mountain – me!) I was desperate for a solution to get my life back. I read books, consumed hundreds of dollars' worth of supplements each month, saw a variety of doctors and healers, tried different types of massage and extremely painful deep-tissue treatments that left me bruised and even tried eating cloves of raw garlic while drinking cabbage juice.

Over the following ten years, chiropractic treatments and massage provided the most relief. One day I said jokingly to my friend, "I should marry a chiropractor; I'm seeing one three times a week!" We both laughed!

I do believe that the universe is listening and knows what we need. Friends set me up on a blind date with a handsome man. Dr. Bruce Nelson was a chiropractor who specialized in chronic pain. I started seeing him professionally, and miracles happened. In just two weeks of treatment with Dr. Bruce I was out of pain, headaches gone, no bowel problems, and I had full range of motion in my neck. My shoulders stopped throbbing, the deep pain in both my arms and hands disappeared, and it no longer felt like I was walking on rocks. I was out of bed early in the morning feeling like I had when I was a kid.

After ten years of constant pain, I was healed. Dr. Bruce not only helped me feel better physically, he healed my broken heart as well. We married that same year and worked side by side for many years. Since we each had six children from our previous marriages, our new family with twelve children made life interesting and joyful, and it still does.

You might be wondering what this story has to do with your challenges with eating. The deeper meaning will help you learn to trust your deepest self and the guidance you are given regarding food. However, before you can discover that meaning, I need to share one more story.

In 2014 Dr. Bruce and I were happily working together helping people with distance energy healing and teaching them the eating techniques you will learn in this book. Our clients were having great results. Our family was doing well and we delighted in our many grandchildren and large family gatherings. Life was very, very good.

In June, three of our active and fun grandsons were at our home for a sleepover. Bruce fixed them their favorite food, pancakes, for dinner that night. All three boys sat around the kitchen counter laughing and singing silly songs with Grandpa Bruce as he flipped pancakes. What a fun evening we had.

Early the next morning while Bruce and I were still in bed, Bruce started clutching his hands to his chest, gurgling, and he was not responsive. I started CPR right away, grabbed the bedside phone, and fumbled with it between chest compressions, finally connecting to 911 on the third try.

My youngest grandson, Hudsen, who was an early riser, peeked into the bedroom. I told him to run fast and wake up his older brother Ayden, who was taller, and tell him to unlock and open the front door and leave it wide open for the ambulance. I ordered the little boys to sit and stay on the living room couch. It seemed like forever before the ambulance arrived. The emergency crew set up their gear as I kept frantically pumping Bruce's chest. They finally placed the defibrillator paddles on his chest and gave him a strong jolt, then lifted his body with the bed sheet and quickly strapped him to a transfer board. The ambulance took Bruce away and I called my daughter Jennifer to come watch the little boys, then jumped out of my nightgown, threw on clothes, and ran out of the house to go to the hospital.

By the time I reached the hospital some of our children had arrived as well as friends and the bishop of our church. Jennifer had called them. We were told that Bruce had experienced a massive aneurysm in his brain and must be airlifted from our home in Montana to Seattle.

All during the flight, I prayed. When we arrived in Seattle, the large emergency room was crowded and overwhelming. Because Bruce's condition was so critical, the doctors could not wait for an operating room. In a non-sterile room with just curtains separating us from the people waiting for treatment, they drilled a hole in his skull to relieve the pressure. I just stood there and prayed. When he was taken for an MRI, I went along, so afraid that if I left his side we'd be separated from each other and I would never see him again. Hours passed and no one knew whether he would live or die.

Bruce miraculously lived. He was in that Seattle hospital for forty-five days. The support we received from family, friends, and total strangers was miraculous. People all over the world prayed for us and sent us love. All twelve of our children, their spouses, and the grandchildren who could, joined us at the hospital with love and support – even one daughter and her husband who lived in South America.

Stress took a terrible toll on me. I was almost out of my mind with worry over how we would ever pay the enormous medical bills, what would happen to the business that Bruce and I shared, and what I would do if Bruce did not recover. My body and mind started to shut down with so much stress. I was barely eating or drinking.

Then I remembered food! I had to start paying attention to my body's needs. I used the techniques in this book to determine what nutrition would support and strengthen me during this stressful time. I also discovered the foods that Bruce needed to encourage healing and worked with the hospital staff to ensure he had them.

His treatment was horrific. He endured multiple surgeries to his brain, tubes in almost every part of his body, and weeks on life support. I spent the weeks wondering if he even knew who I was. He had to relearn how to swallow, control his bowel and bladder, walk, talk, and everything else. Thankfully he does not remember most of his time in the hospital. I do. The nurses cautioned me that relatives often end up in worse shape than the person in the hospital. Without my faith, the support we received, and my knowledge of how to nurture myself with good food and nutrition, I would not have been able to cope.

Today Bruce and I are doing well although both of us needed over two years to recover. Our healing processes were, and continue to be, supported by the foods our bodies tell us we need.

There are challenges and stress in your life. They may be different from what I experienced but they can cause you to feel depleted and to have challenges with your health or weight. Whether you are experiencing health problems or are underweight or overweight, your body is asking you for the foods it needs to heal. You might feel a strange hunger or have a strong desire for certain foods at times. This is your body's wisdom whispering to you and nudging you. Your body's wisdom is perfect for you and available at any time. Let me show you how to access it!

CHAPTER 2
Why Diets Don't Work

If you have formed the habit of checking on every new diet that comes along, you will find that, mercifully, they all blur together, leaving you with only one definite piece of information: French-fried potatoes are out.
– Jean Kerr

When I was in my mid-thirties, I had some serious trouble with irritable bowel and digestion. I read about the power of juicing. This was long before it was popular, and it was considered by almost everyone I knew to be a weird treatment, just for health nuts. I surmised from my reading that garlic and cabbage were good for the digestion, so I borrowed a juicer from a friend and juiced a huge head of cabbage. Then I popped a big fresh clove of garlic in my mouth, chewed it up, and gulped down a very large glass of green cabbage juice. It came right back up and I felt worse than ever! I did not know about the Food Codes.

How many diets have you tried? Some diets are scientifically researched; some are just plain crazy! There's the all-egg diet, the lemonade cleanse, the oatmeal diet, low fat, high fat, low carb, all carb, no sugar… the list of crazy diets is endless. We all want to know what the perfect diet is and what foods will help us have trim and healthy bodies. But there is not one single diet that fills this bill... until now!

Just as each person's fingerprints are different, so are each person's nutritional needs and solutions. You have your own unique health issues, and foods that are healing and health-building for one person can cause another person great distress, such as pain, inflammation, bloating, weight problems, allergies, and even disease. Whether you are overweight, underweight, or lacking energy, your relationship with food is personal and unique to you.

The word *diet* is one of the most misused words in our language today. It is associated with restriction, starvation, dread, pain, and suffering, yet is what we think we must endure to be the thin, willowy figures society paints for us as pictures of happiness and fulfillment. It's used like a swear word. The D-word conjures the dreadful act of self-depravation and stress that 108 million Americans attempt four or five times each year. The diet industry currently rakes in over $66 billion a year.

You've seen the success testimonies that accompany diet programs that have come down the pike. At the end of every TV diet commercial or magazine ad featuring a skinny model prancing around half naked in a bikini, is the tiny statement *Results Not Typical.

Typical diet programs are based on restrictions – some that are just crazy and dangerous. They usually limit the dieter to tiny portions; restrict calories, carbohydrates, sugar, and/or fat; and regulate specific foods. It's a mindset of all or nothing: When you are not dieting, you can eat *all* that you want; when you are on a diet, you can eat "nothing." This is where the term "yoyo dieting" comes from. You might go on a strict diet to lose weight for a wedding, a class reunion, or to look good in a swimsuit while on vacation, and gain the weight back right afterward. You might get good results from a diet once but fail miserably the next time you try it. Why is that? You will learn the answer in this book.

It can be so confusing to know what to eat for good health. One expert tells you to eat fish and olive oil. Another says green juices. In 2017 *U. S. News & World Report* reported on the top thirty-eight diets... the top thirty-eight out of how many? Goodness, thirty-eight is a *lot* of diets! It seems like every few months a different food will either cure you or kill you.

I used to own a health food store. When customers came in and asked for no-fat products, I joked that someday lard would be the next fad food – that we'd have lard capsules in the store and people would buy them in droves. Guess what? Lard can be a healthy and useful food for some people, at least according to an article by Pete Wells published in 2012 in *Food and Wine* magazine entitled "Lard: The New Heath Food?"

In fact, there was a recent world summit at which scientists said they had been wrong about fat; that it is essential for good health; and that butter, coconut oil, and other fats should be consumed regularly. Lard and animal fat have been attacked as unhealthy foods for decades. We were told they clog our arteries and lead to heart attack and death. And now lard is being heralded as a health food. No wonder we don't know what to eat!

The abundance of food available to Americans today has never been equaled. Food is everywhere and is prepackaged for instant consumption. This is a luxurious convenience, yet there are an increasing number of added chemicals in our foods. Many of us no longer eat the same whole, natural foods that were readily available when we were children.

Let's consider the original meaning of the word *diet*. Its first known use was in the thirteenth century and was based on the Latin word *diaeta*, meaning "regimen." *Diet* truly means a manner of living that includes the food we eat and the way we eat it. My purpose in writing this book is to show you how to use food as a source of health, healing, joy, and satisfaction for a great lifestyle.

Instead of causing you guilt and confusion I'll show you how to take the stress out of the D-word lifestyle. I'll show you how to determine what is good for your body to eat so that you will no longer be at the mercy of the latest fad diet or new expert touting a theory. Using the Food Codes provides a harmonious relationship with yourself, your food, and the world. It doesn't get any better than that!

Joann's Story

When we met, Joann, who was in her fifties, called herself the Queen of Dieting, as she had tried diets, exercise, and coaching and was still trying every diet that came across her path. She was depressed and obsessed with being thin. She was exhausted even though she slept a lot, and her career as a college professor was on the line. Joann was thin – what some would call skinny, and she looked gaunt.

Her mother was a very tiny woman at 4 feet 9 inches and 94 pounds, and by the age of twelve Joann was the same height and weight as her mother. Joann's weight was average for a child her age, but she felt big and fat. She was constantly compared to her very petite cousin, and she was teased and called fat by her brothers. Her mother closely watched what Joann ate and scolded her if she thought she was eating too much. Joann's self-esteem was so low that she would sneak food and eat it where no one could see her.

Joann said that all she could see when she looked in the mirror, even as an adult, was the girl who was always bigger than her mother and her cousin. Joann counted calories and carbs for everything she ate and avoided fat like the plague. She had been on a raw diet and juicing for seven months wondering when her energy level was going to rise. When Joann and I developed her Food Codes food plan, it showed that she needed chicken and chicken fat for key proteins. She laughed because her Jewish grandmother's Sunday chicken soup made with *schmaltz* (chicken fat) was her favorite food! Her grandmother spread the creamy *schmaltz* on toast like butter for Joann. White fish also tested as a great protein for Joann. This made her laugh too! She also loved her grandmother's gefilte fish, another Jewish dish. (Her brothers hated it.) Her Food Codes plan included a nice variety of vegetables and fermented foods; a few fruits; and various grains, nuts, and seeds. She needed 50 percent cooked food and 50 percent raw food. Her greens needed to be steamed or cooked rather than raw, and she needed no green juice at that time.

Ten years later Joann is feeling good about herself. She left her college career for a while but is now teaching again. We helped clear her struggle with childhood emotional issues and she now uses the Food Codes method to test what foods her body needs and wants. I recently saw her, and as she brushed her hands down her hips and lovingly patted her belly, she said, "Look at this beautiful belly. It's not caved in any more. My body loves me, and I love my body." Joann is about fifteen pounds heavier than she was when we first met, and this is exactly what her body wants.

CHAPTER 3

Understanding Food's Role

What is food to one person, is to others bitter poison.
– Titus Lucretius Carus (96–55 BC)

"Eat this, it's good for you." "Don't eat that, it's bad for you." You hear these statements all the time. But how can you really know what's "good" for you and what's "bad" for you? We love to eat, and more than that we have to eat. Food, air, and water are primary requirements to sustain life.

Food news is major news these days. Pesticides and chemicals, processed foods, salt, sugar, bad fats, good fats, organic, not organic, GMO, BHA, BHT, and GRAS – yikes! What does it all mean? (GRAS stands for Generally Recognized as Safe, a term thrown out to cover the producer's backside when a GRAS food is later reported to cause cancer!) Just when we feel comfortable with the way our refrigerators are stocked some news flash blurts out, "Don't eat that!"

Amid all this controversy and conflicting information, only you, armed with the knowledge of how food really works and your highest inner wisdom, can determine what should you ingest. You'll never again feel confused about what to eat or drink. Let's start with how food impacts you and your health.

What Are the Food Codes?

Deoxyribonucleic acid, or DNA, is the molecule in each cell that contains and carries instructions to the cells used in the reproduction, growth, development, and functioning of all humans, animals, plants, and living things – called the *genetic code*. There is a popular saying that humans and bananas share 50 percent of their DNA. Does that mean we are half related to a banana? No – even if you have a family member who is quite slippery. What sharing 50 percent of our DNA with a banana really means is that both humans and bananas have many of the same particular genes that code for certain functions, such as cell growth.

All DNA is a code consisting of four letters: A, C, G, and T, which stand for adenine, cytosine, guanine, and thymine. They are the building blocks that code for the amino acids all proteins are made of. All living things share the same basic genes. What makes humans different from animals and plants is the order in which these basic genes are organized and when they are activated, called *sequencing*. That difference in order and activation is what creates each individual living thing, from a banana to a fruit fly to a human.

It is amazing that we share DNA with all living things, including all foods from living sources. This is likely the reason why whole, living foods are so important for our health and healing. Even though they share the same basic DNA, each individual plant and animal food vibrates with the energy of its own individual frequency that I call its Food Code. Your body is a vessel of vibrating energy, requiring consumption of the best energy available from food, air, water, and sunlight, if you desire the most energetic body possible. When consumed, this energy actually becomes your body. "You are what you eat" is true.

I will show you how to test each food's code – or energy – to determine what foods are best for your body.

Gary's Story

In the past several months I have made more lasting, positive changes in my life than I have in the past ten years. I have tried many different modalities and only had little to no success in releasing stuck energies and emotions. Some would last for a few weeks maybe, but then would return as if I had done nothing at all. With the help of Lana and her expertise in the use of the Body Code and Emotion Code work, I have cleared many emotional blockages and holding patterns. When Lana offered to help me with a food list, it was a no-brainer for me.

I have been eating mostly what I want when I want with little to no effect that I have ever noticed (so I thought). That does not mean that I was not having reactions to the food I was eating, it just means I was not sensitive enough to notice them. With the work I previously received from the Body Code and the Emotion Code I have also become more sensitive to what I put in my body. Some of the items on the Food Codes Food List that I should avoid caught me by surprise, like bananas, table salt, stevia, popcorn and peanut butter. Some of these were my favorites!

I took to my new food plan with excitement in figuring out just how good I could feel. If it was anything like I experienced with my other session with Lana, it was going to be amazing! For the past two-and-a-half months I have been following my list of approved and not approved food items. Some foods have been harder than others to not use like coffee, white sugar, and table salt. I can say that the changes I feel now are well worth it. Things like gas, bloating, low energy, stomach aches and indigestion have all improved significantly and some are completely gone. Now when I cheat and add these items back into my diet, I notice the effects within hours and feel the after effects for hours or days.

One thing I was not expecting was having a decrease in my overall body aches and pains. I was hard on myself as a young man and my almost thirteen years in the military did not do me any good either. I was starting to accept the fact that I was just going to have to live with my aches and pains as part of paying the price. With my changes in my food, using the Food Codes plan provided to me by Lana, I have noticed a decrease in aches, pains, and swelling. So thinking I was able to eat almost anything without repercussion was not true. I now can see and feel the effects on my body.

I say thank you to Lana for showing me a way to eat that was not out of some cook book or diet plan, but rather a plan designed for me, energetically by me. No diet, food, or any other system I tried felt right or energetically pleasing. This has been all of that and I get to eat many things that other diets would forbid. This does not feel like a diet at all but rather a lifestyle choice. So thank you, Lana, and I look forward to my adjusted food plans moving forward to see how they change and grow for me.

The Food Pyramid

A lot of people look at good eating as just good common sense. The question that is apparent, though, is what information that "good common sense" is based on.

It started with the food pyramid, which made "good common sense" to many people partly because it was well promoted, put constantly in front of us for years, and became familiar to us. It was originally a pyramid-shaped diagram divided into food-group sections to show the recommended food intake for each food group. The first food pyramid was published in Sweden in 1974. The most widely known food pyramid was introduced by the United States Department of Agriculture in 1992 under the name Food Guide Pyramid, was updated in 2005, and then replaced by MyPlate in 2011. Over twenty-five other countries and organizations have published their own food pyramids.

The newest food guide from the USDA is MyPlate, which looks like a dinner plate divided into four colored sections labeled "Fruits," "Grains," "Proteins," and "Vegetables," with a circle next to it depicting a glass with the label "Dairy." The USDA has a new interactive website, ChooseMyPlate.gov, that promotes a lot of ideas about food and how to better use foods for health.

A food guide is a good idea and is intended to help, yet there really is no way to apply the Food Guide Pyramid, MyPlate, or whatever the idea may morph into, to the mass public. It is difficult to assess what is good for you individually from what is thought to be good for everyone in general. Regardless of how the pyramid is stacked, or the plate arranged, each individual should eat according to their body's current needs. There is no "one size fits all" with food!

In my many years of helping people with their nutritional needs, I've observed that our bodies and our energy are in constant motion trying to maintain balance within our environment. The weather, our stress level, and our general health all impact what we need. No general food guide can adequately address those constant changes.

According to the World Health Organization's website, "Health is more than the absence of disease. Health is a state of optimal well-being." My definition of *vibrant health* is a radiance of peace and a calm centeredness inside you in the midst of whatever is happening in the world outside. Balance is at the center of this. Good nutrition is a large part of achieving balance, and whole foods are at the center of good nutrition. Good food is at the core of good health.

We are living in a world today where lemonade is made from artificial flavors and furniture polish is made from real lemons.
– Alfred E. Newman

Glossary of Common Food Labels

Back in Grandma's day food was food. Today food is labeled. Terms like *whole foods, organic foods,* and *GMOs* are tossed around so frequently that we don't want to look stupid by admitting we don't know exactly what they mean. Here are some of these terms defined:

Whole Foods

Whole foods are not created in a laboratory. They generally do not come in a box with a long list of ingredients on the side label. They don't have to be organic, locally grown, or free from pesticides; they are simply complete foods without adding anything to them. An orange is a whole food while a glass of orange juice is not. An egg is a whole food while an egg white is not. They are in their natural, unchanged state.

Several whole foods combined together, for example, an omelet using whole eggs, sliced mushrooms, cherry tomatoes, sliced onions, and fresh basil leaf, are also considered whole foods.

Whole foods contain whole nutrition. They contain the exact nutrition in the exact proportions intended by nature for that particular food. When you think of whole foods you probably think of fruits like apples, oranges, bananas; vegetables like carrots, potatoes, and zucchini; and maybe eggs, grains, and beans. How about meats and fish? The last time many of us had whole meat was at Thanksgiving dinner when the head of the household cut the turkey off of the bone (though it might have had flavors and preservatives injected into it). Most of the chicken available at grocery stores is now skinless and boneless. Most of the beef, lamb, pork, and fish are also boneless because we want more convenience with our fast-paced lives, and trimmed of fat because we have been trained to fear fat. I don't consider those whole foods because without the skin, bone, and fat they lose some of the nutrition that makes them truly whole foods.

Red meat is not bad for you.
Now blue-green meat, that's bad for you!
– Tommy Smothers

We have been taught to fear whole-fat dairy foods. Many studies showed that full-fat organic dairy products were wholesome foods; and pasteurization has come under scrutiny after some studies found it reduced nutritional content. In European countries where full-fat and raw dairy milk are the norm, there is less heart disease than we experience in America.

The more healthy, whole foods you eat, the easier it is for your body to maintain itself and build new cells to replace the millions of body cells that die every day. A house built with pieces and parts of low-quality building products will not stand the tests of structural stress nor last as long as a house that is built with the highest grade and quality building materials. It makes sense that whole foods make better body-building materials. By adding to your diet more of the whole foods that test good for you using the Food Codes method, there is a very good chance you will be able to eat your way out of any dilemma you are in, be it poor health, overweight, skin conditions, or lack of vitality.

For example, raw honey, which is a whole food, is a healthier sweetener than white sugar, which is processed and refined. The nutrients found in whole foods are highly complex structures that combine a variety of known and yet-to-be-discovered elements all working together. This enables the food to do the best job of healthy cell-building in your body. Scientists are discovering new nutritional elements in food on a regular basis. I relate this process to discovering, after eons of believing the world to be flat and the center of the universe, that not only is the world round but there are unnumbered worlds far out in space.

Nutrients from a whole food cannot be taken apart or isolated from the whole and do the same job as the complete whole food. The nutrients in each food are created to work in a specific synergy, all parts working together.

Processed Foods

Throughout history it has been necessary to preserve foods in ways that extend their storage life. Through the ages man has dried, frozen, fermented, cured, smoked, and salted foods to preserve them for later use. This was the first form of processed food. Processed foods are foods that have been modified from their original whole form by man. This process changes the structure and the vibrational energy of the original food. There are many diverse reasons for the evolution of modern processed food in our Western culture, and there are many books and documentaries available on this subject with ideas ranging from the growing population to conspiracy theories.

Huge grocery stores have replaced local markets because they can distribute more food in large urban areas. There is also an ever-increasing variety of foods from other countries available due to new preserving techniques, packaging methods, and shipping practices. Food stores are glutted with new packaged food products and continually changing and expanding product lines.

According to the Academy of Nutrition and Dietetics (AND), there is a spectrum of food processing:

Minimally Processed Foods – like bagged spinach, cut vegetables and roasted nuts, are often simply pre-prepped for convenience. These types of foods need to be processed at their peak of ripeness or freshness to lock in nutritional quality and freshness. Examples of foods to be frozen or canned are beans and tomatoes, other fruits and vegetables, including canned tuna and fish.

Peak processed foods are usually canned, dried or frozen. The actual end nutrition values and quality of the individual food can vary from each individual food and with the canning, freezing or drying process. The type of container and what it is made from can make a difference with how healthy the food is and how long it will last, even though vegetables, fruits and meats are processed at their peak of freshness.

[The] list of Minimally Processed Foods also includes milk and dairy or cultured foods like yogurt, sour cream and cultured vegetables such as sauerkraut and kimchi. Some natural nut butters fall in this category. Frozen French fry potatoes, burger patties and other lightly processed meats etc. are categorized as peak to minimally processed. Peak processed foods may have added salt, sugar or oils but usually a very short list of additives.

(http://msue.anr.msu.edu/news/what_is_a_processed_food)

I am not suggesting that all food processing is bad or unhealthy. Minimally processed whole foods like bags of baby carrots, vegetables, combination veggie trays, and bagged salads and greens are acceptable and convenient ways to get your fresh veggies and fruits. Again, from the AND spectrum:

More to Most Processed Added Ingredient Foods – Foods with ingredients added for flavor and texture (such as sweeteners, spices, oils, colors and preservatives) include jarred pasta sauce, salad dressing, yogurt and readymade mixes. Ready-to-eat foods, like crackers, cereals, and deli meat, are more heavily processed. The most heavily processed foods often are frozen or pre-made meals like frozen pizza and microwaveable dinners. These next levels of foods with added ingredients can vary from a few ingredients to many. These are foods in which raw ingredients have been transformed into something new and different. This is where the water gets murky real fast and there is no drawing a defined line. It is difficult to list categories of foods here aside from saying that this category contains anything with a label of over five ingredients, whether boxed, canned, bagged, dried, frozen or other. These are the foods found on the inside shelf area of your grocery store.

(http://msue.anr.msu.edu/news/what_is_a_processed_food)

Note that the foods in this category include organic processed foods and foods that claim to be "100% Natural." Organic processed foods are still processed foods no matter how much better it makes you feel to buy organic. Organic sugar is still sugar. The word *natural* on a food label is subject to definitions that keep changing with labeling laws. The lists of ingredients in these foods are just as long as they are for other processed, packaged foods.

Enriched Foods

Foods that are labeled "enriched" have had nutrients added to them to replace those lost during processing. For example, when whole wheat is milled into white flour, the nutritious germ and bran and the vitamins, minerals, micronutrients, and fiber they contain are stripped away and lost. White flour and white flour products were some of the first foods to be enriched and fortified in the advent of food processing companies. Many of the nutrients added to enriched foods are manufactured in laboratories.

Fortified Foods

You've seen commercials touting orange juice with added calcium and cereals with added vitamins. Those foods are fortified by adding extra nutrients such as vitamins and minerals that may or may not have been originally present in the food.

Enriching and fortifying foods sound like good ideas, right? The nutrients that have been stripped out are added back, or more nutrients are added to make it even better. This solution, though, is like someone who has stolen thousands of dollars from you compensating you by giving you back a few pennies or paying you in Monopoly Money. That is not very "enriching," and adding back chemically synthesized nutrients can't make up for stealing a food's natural micronutrients. Again, most nutrients used to fortify foods are synthesized in laboratories.

The list of fortified foods grows daily and includes breakfast cereals, snack foods, desserts, and vitamin waters. The massive explosion of fortified foods has resulted in the use of the term *functional foods*, which mean they are formulated for a specific purpose or task. New York University Hospital physician Dr. Mark Siegel was interviewed on the subject of food fortifying and said his concern was that people would eat more fortified foods thinking they were getting health benefits when the foods themselves were unhealthy. Is cereal with yogurt bits in it healthier than cereal without them? No; it's just an advertising scam. There is no yogurt in that cereal, just sugary bits of added chemicals.

Food fortification was implemented by the World Health Organization (WHO) and the Food and Agricultural Organization (FAO) of the US. They wanted to help decrease nutritional deficiencies on a global level. The first foods targeted for fortification were milk and milk products, fats and oils, infant formulas, teas, and beverages.

Food fortification is not just about quantifying nutrients though; it's about ethics. Human rights issues have been broached by fortifying food, even though the WHO was key in implementing the practice. The WHO states that customers have the right to choose whether or not they want fortified food products, but when legislation was passed that mandated fortifying certain foods, that choice was taken away. Fortifying foods also makes them cost more, which can keep the target market, the underprivileged, from being able to buy them.

> *We may find in the long run that tinned food is a deadlier weapon than the machine gun.*
> *– George Orwell*

GMOs

Genetically Modified Organisms (GMOs) are organisms that have specific changes made to their DNA using methods of genetic engineering. Foods with these organisms engineered into them are often called "GMO foods" though the proper term is *genetically modified foods*, or *GM foods*. The Flavr Savr tomato was introduced in 1994. This genetically modified tomato was engineered to delay the ripening process to withstand a longer transit time before ripening. Tomatoes have also been engineered for tougher skin to withstand shipping with less damage. Most food engineering efforts have been aimed at cash crops like soy beans, corn, canola/rapeseed, and cotton seed. Genetically modified livestock are being experimentally developed. This sounds like science fiction, but it is really happening.

A lot of controversy surrounds the creating and farming of GM foods. Concerns center on the safety of humans and animals eating these foods and environmental concerns. Many people are concerned that GM seeds and animals may be subject to intellectual property rights owned by multinational corporations. They are worried about the effect of GM foods on our health and environment, as well as the implications of government regulation and control over them.

Organic Foods

Organic foods are grown without using chemical fertilizers and growth agents. Until the twentieth century all food grown worldwide was organic. Our ancestors ate completely organic diets. Modern farming today uses many chemicals to produce food. These chemicals are absorbed by foods and by soil and water.

"Know your farmer, know your food" became the motto of an initiative instituted by the USDA in September of 2009. The US, Canada, and other countries have developed regulations to support organic farming practices. The US is currently importing large amounts of organic foods from foreign countries to meet the demand of American consumers.

The certified organic food industry in the US is currently a $50 billion industry. *The Washington Post* and other news sources have exposed some big food companies in the US that are selling "organic" foods that actually are not. Such articles also warn of other fraud in the industry, some even questioning the reliability of the USDA organic seal. A $90 billion industry of products sold as "natural," "all natural," and "100% natural," is an even bigger group reported to be perpetrating labeling and marketing fraud. Consumer confidence has been badly undermined by these controversies. One concerned writer mentioned that after reading a May 2017 article in *The Washington Post* by Peter Whoriskey called "Why Your 'Organic' Milk May Not Be Organic," you might wonder if you are being scammed all the time.

It was a real novelty when organic candy arrived at my health food store. We put out a sample basket of wrapped candy drops. Mothers would marvel at organic candies and treats and were much more likely to let their kids have them than other treats. The organic gummy bears were colored with food dyes like beet juice rather than manufactured dyes. The M&M-like candies with organic chocolate and sugar were huge sellers. Customers came in daily for the big organic cookies we carried and an organic sugar-sweetened drink for their breaks. The organic Oreo-like cookies were hot items for the health food junkies.

The debate about whether organic foods are better for us than conventional foods is heated and complex. There are studies that showed there were virtually no differences in the quality of the two types of foods, while other studies showed that organic food is more nutritious. Documentaries have been produced showing the benefits of organic farming, but others have been produced that exposed farmers who claimed organic practices that were found to be grossly fraudulent. Some farmers who claimed to raise chickens organically actually raised them in the same horrible conditions in which some conventional farmers do.

Food goes through a lot to end up on our hometown grocery shelves. Some travels around the globe to get to us; it wasn't picked fresh yesterday. Organic foods also make a journey through many hands and venders to get to market. How fresh or safe any food *really* is, is a quandary. There is no way for consumers to know exactly what foods have gone through to reach our grocery stores or what human, rodent, insect, or contaminant might have affected it along the way. Which shopper just fingered the food or sprayed the produce isle with a germ-filled sneeze? Does this sound like an overwhelming dilemma? (You *can* know what the best food is for you by using the testing technique I will teach you in later chapters.)

Leigh's Story

My family and I used to eat out of the box or eat out for almost every meal. We have gradually become health conscious with more and more information available in the news about food, diets, and what we should and should not eat. I follow some really good food and eating blogs but sometimes they have conflicting opinions about food.

With what I've learned about food and nutrition, I worked up to buying mostly organic foods and I have weaned my family away from eating the regular packaged foods that used to be the biggest part of our diet. I learned the Food Codes food-testing technique and started using it to test the foods I buy in the grocery store when I go shopping. I was really surprised when I found that organic food did not always test as the best food to buy. Sometimes the regular food would test higher, like nonorganic apples over organic apples.

I thought I was doing something wrong and that my testing was not accurate. With continued experience using the Food Codes method to do my grocery shopping, I find that my testing really is very accurate. Sometimes the nonorganic apples just are better quality than the organic ones. I don't know why, and I really don't need to know why. I am grateful to be able to test what foods and products are best for me and my family.

By using the Food Codes method, I feel that we are eating healthier now than we ever have. This gives me confidence as a mom knowing that I am feeding my family the best foods. My teenaged son has learned the Food Codes testing and it has made him more aware of healthy food choices when he eats out and with his friends.

The Food Codes testing technique is very simple, fast, and discrete. Individual foods vary in quality. Organic produce is best only about half the time. Locally grown food tests high most of the time, and of course it is always much fresher. However, there is more to good nutrition than just understanding food labels and eating well. Did you know that your emotions can impact the positive benefits of the food you eat? Turn the page and find out how even the best food can't heal a totally stressed-out body.

CHAPTER 4

The Impact of Emotions on Your Weight, Food, and How You Eat It

Worries go down better with soup.
– Jewish proverb

Weight problems often have little to do with the food you're eating and more to do with how you feel. We've all experienced food cravings. When we see something upsetting on television, feel angry or bored, or have had a rough day, we soothe ourselves with something sweet, crunchy, or creamy. Whether you turn to ice cream, candy, crackers, or chips, you know what it's like to use food to heal a painful emotion. Then there is the bingeing hangover – the feelings of disgust, judgment, and shame in regard to what you just splurged on, that make you feel even worse than before you put that first morsel into your mouth.

Emotions strongly impact our eating and our cravings. When we release some of the stress, guilt, and drama in our lives, we find more balance in our eating – we are drawn to foods that are better for us, eat only when hungry, and stop eating when full. We find true joy and peace in eating and food, as the Creator intended.

Emotional imbalances can be 85 to 95 percent of our eating and weight struggles. We unknowingly hold on to our emotions at a subconscious level where they can affect our eating without our realizing it. Emotions can cause pain and discomfort in many ways, including food cravings and eating disorders. The emotions trapped in your subconscious can actually take up space in your body. The result can be pain, eating disorders, and being overweight or underweight, among other problems.

<u>Michael Pollan</u> wrote in his book *In Defense of Food: An Eater's Manifesto,* about a man who "showed the words 'chocolate cake' to a group of Americans and recorded their word associations. 'Guilt' was the top response. If that strikes you as unexceptional, consider the response of French eaters to the same prompt: 'celebration.'"

Your cravings can provide clues about what your body needs. If you are drawn to cheese crackers or cheese puffs, your body might need more dairy products. Cravings for potato chips can signal a desire for salt to boost the power of your adrenal glands. The smooth, creamy texture of ice cream might remind you of childhood days when you were comforted by your mother and the fizz and sweetness of soda pop might remind you of the special, fun treat soda was when you went on a family trip. It is almost impossible to separate a food craving from an underlying emotion.

Since we're considering emotions, we should also consider relationships in regard to eating habits. Your first two relationships on this planet were with your mother and with food. You are probably aware of the effects of your relationship with your mother on your life, whether or not it was a loving relationship; but what impact has your relationship with food had on your life? Ponder that for a moment.

Patty's Story

Patty had been plagued with digestive issues for over a year, and she had gained a lot of weight. On a recent trip to see her family she was miserable with pain and bloating and ate antacids "like a kid with a bag of jelly beans." She called and asked if I could help. I used a technique called the Emotion Code, developed by Dr. Bradley Nelson, my brilliant brother-in-law. The Emotion Code teaches how to find and release trapped emotions. I used this technique to help Patty.

What I found bothering Patty's digestion, and particularly her liver, was an emotion of frustration. She knew immediately where this emotion came from. About a year earlier her husband had been promoted at work. Patty was not happy about it because this promotion took him out of town for most of the week; she had her own job and needed help with the kids. She said she had felt constant frustration with all she had on her plate during the past year. She had grabbed many meals on the go and had not been eating right.

As Patty cleared the emotion of frustration, she had the strangest feeling. "My belly has been so bloated, and now it feels like a big beach ball with the air hissing out." Her abdomen felt lighter and lighter, and suddenly her pants didn't feel as tight. We were both pretty amazed.

I helped Patty clear some other emotions and we tested a Food Codes plan for her that she has used to find the best foods to eat at home and at restaurants. She dropped four pounds the first week and continued toward her goal weight. Her digestion quieted down and she kicked the antacids. She felt much happier with her husband and her kids after the emotional clearing and stopped eating in front of the TV in the evening.

Stress Can Make You Fat and Sick

General stress coupled with emotional stress is associated with innumerable problems including being overweight and underweight. And eating food that is not right for you causes you more stress! Accumulated stress overloads the body and is the beginning of all disease.

Vi and Bob's Story

My husband retired from a very busy law practice at age seventy. I thought we would be having more fun after he retired, but Bob was too tired to do much. Every morning Bob would eat his usual cereal and toast piled with jam for breakfast, get up from the table, and have to go lie back down for an hour or two. He would have to nap after lunch, also. Bob's doctor said he just needed to lose weight due to his high blood pressure and constant fatigue.

I had had some health problems several years ago and Lana really helped me get healthy. I loved the food plan she gave me as part of my treatment program. I found out that many of the foods I ate all the time were causing me problems. When I started eating the food on my plan, I had a lot more energy and no more digestive problems.

Bob supports me in my natural healing and health ideas, but he eats as he pleases. He loves bread, cheese, and ice cream. When he finally agreed to have a food plan tested, guess what foods were causing him to be so tired? You guessed it: bread, cheese, and ice cream. The yeast in bread was bothering him and so were dairy products.

Through testing Bob's Food Codes, we found some alternatives to dairy products and natural yeast bread that tested good for Bob. He replaced dairy with coconut milk and almond milk. He loves coconut-milk ice cream even more than he loved dairy ice cream and has a small bowl now and then. We found that sourdough bread was a good food for Bob. Lana brought us a loaf of her homemade sourdough bread and Bob was in heaven. He stopped eating cheese for several weeks, and in testing a new food plan later we found that he can now eat a certain kind of cheese with no problems. Using the Food Codes plan has made Bob much more aware of his food choices and it has helped me to know what to cook for us both.

Bob lost his tiredness, and he lost fifteen pounds when he started eating the foods that are good for him, and he gained his energy back. We are going on a long-dreamed-about trip and we will be gone for several months. I am glad to have a husband who has energy to travel and have fun with.

Food can be such a pleasurable experience. We really love to eat. You might not have thought of food as a stressor before, but here is some food for thought: The last two decades have produced a large amount of research that linked stress to obesity and diseases such as diabetes, autoimmune diseases, fibromyalgia, chronic fatigue, and many other conditions and diseases. Increased fat-storing, abdominal obesity, low metabolism, high blood sugar, and hormone problems are all linked to stress. To understand how to be slim and trim or how to heal and be well, it is important to first understand the body and the stress process that wears the body down.

It's probably hard for you to remember the last time you had forty-eight hours of peace with time for meditation or just relaxing and feeling happy and content; but it's probably easy to remember the last time you experienced something stressful like rushing to get ready for work and get your kids off to school, a deadline at work, or an argument with someone. Stress is a natural reaction in humans and animals. The key word is *reaction*. Each person reacts differently to that which they perceive as stress. Some people are very sensitive to changes in the energy around them. What is a grievous stressor to one person, might not bother another person at all.

Psychologist Richard Lazarus refers to stress as any event in which environmental demands, internal demands, or both tax or exceed an individual's adaptive resources. If your life seems calm and normal, you might think your psychological stress is low, but dieting, overexercising, insomnia, infections, poor dental hygiene, environmental toxins, and even the political situation, can be causing you subconscious stress.

Your body can handle acute or short-term stress quite well and recover from it, but you are not built to handle the chronic, unrelenting stress so rampant in our society today. Dr. Peter Levine said that our stress response is designed to last about forty-five seconds, not twenty-four hours, or day after day.

Constant stress causes the body to be "turned on" all the time, and not in a good way. The sympathetic nervous system, which stimulates bodily functions, goes haywire and the adrenal system gets stuck in the "fight, flight, or freeze" response. These systems stay turned on like a car alarm constantly blaring in the background.

The adrenal glands are small, triangular endocrine glands that sit on top of the kidneys, waiting patiently to be called to duty. Their major role is to release hormones like cortisol and adrenaline in response to stress.

Stress activates or depresses several functions in the body. Digestion is halted. The hypothalamus gland signals the adrenal system, and the sympathetic nervous system shoots impulses through the body. The heart beats faster, muscles tense, eyes dilate, and the mouth gets dry. This reaction has been named the *fight or flight response*. The body can't tell the difference between being chased by a tiger or getting stuck in traffic; it just senses stress and kicks into gear.

Beyond fight and flight there is a third reaction to stress: freeze. Your body can stop you right in your tracks like a deer in the headlights. An overwhelming trauma can instantly stun you with a wave of hopelessness when it appears you have no chance for conquest or escape. Your blood pressure quickly drops when you freeze, and you can fall or faint. The parasympathetic branch of the nervous system, which calms you down to rest and digest, clamps down and takes over from the freeze response.

Any way your body deals with stress, whether it be fight, flight, or freeze, halts your digestive system. Stress can make you sick and fat, and the food you eat might be doing no good for you at all.

> *Ask not what you can do for your country.*
> *Ask what's for lunch.*
> *– Orson Wells*

Stress can be real and tangible, or imagined. Imagined stress causes worry. Your body reacts to worry in the same way it does to actual stressful situations.

There is good stress and bad stress. Good stress, called eustress, is caused by things like buying a new house, getting married, and going to a party. You process good stress in the same way as the bad stress I discussed above.

What about guilt? Ever beat yourself up for how you look or what you eat? Ever compare yourself to others and feel ugly? Thinking negatively about your appearance, eating patterns, or weight adds an additional load of stress and sends you scurrying for a glass of wine or a jumbo order of nachos.

Conditions in our environment can be stressful on the body, too, such as the changing of the season. Heat and cold can create stress, whether you're indoors or out. Your body has different requirements for food in the hot summertime than it does in the cold of winter. Your body probably needs light, cooling foods in the summer, like fruits, vegetables, and raw foods, and requires less food than at other times of the year. If you live where the winters are cold, your body needs complex or concentrated foods that create heat in the winter, like meats, grains, and beans. And you might need to eat more food in the winter than in the summer.

Your body's nutritional requirements change with any number of different kinds of stresses in your life. Studies have shown that diet helps or hinders your stress load depending on the type of nutrition you take in. Food that has been healthy for you in the past can become unhealthy for you, and vice versa. This can be due to changes in your body from reactions to stress, health conditions, aging, and a list of other factors that can be summed up in one word: *anything*. And your life is constantly changing. It's different than it was five years ago, and probably five months ago or even five days ago.

Stress affects your entire energetic being and bringing your energy back into balance can require a particular food. The only way to determine what your body needs to enjoy balance is to ask it using the Food Codes method.

Robyn's Story

The Food Codes food plan has helped me to feel more energized and clearheaded. Using my good foods I felt more energized and alert. The food plan also helped to support my body while it was in the process of healing. I had just started Body Code sessions with Lana to address a chronic stress issue, and I feel the food plan helped my body heal and recover faster. I felt a tangible improvement in my condition after about two-and-a-half weeks.

Having this knowledge empowers us to take control of our own healing. It's amazing to have this tool available to us. It allows us to tailor our food intake to exactly what our bodies need at the moment. It takes a lot of the guesswork out of figuring out what our bodies need to heal and become stronger. Thank you, Lana, for developing this amazing tool!

Energy and Balance

A balanced diet is a cookie in each hand.
– Barbara Jonson

The Food Codes use the energy of food to balance the energetic body you live in. Einstein said that everything is energy. We learned in science class that everything in nature is vibrating energy. The atoms and molecules of every kind of substance vibrate with energy frequencies. The desk you sit at appears solid but is actually vibrating with energy, though it is moving at such a low speed that it appears to be totally solid. Sound has such a high vibration that we can't see it, and some frequencies of sound vibrate at such a high speed that we can't hear them.

The earth has a magnetic, vibrating energy field. Your body is also made up of vibrating energy frequencies. Every organ and gland has its own particular frequency of vibration. The term *energy field* is used to describe the energy around an object. Your body is pure energy and has an electromagnetic energy field. The energy field of your body can be detected and measured from several feet away.

The parts of your body are interconnected in very complex ways right down to the subatomic level. For thousands of years scientists and healers have told us of this incredible connection between our physical, mental, emotional, and spiritual dimensions. Just as you have unique fingerprints, your energetic vibration is also unique to you.

When your body is vibrating at its optimal frequency and you are balanced physically, mentally, emotionally, and spiritually, you are healthy. When your body is not balanced energetically it is not as healthy and cannot function harmoniously. The Food Codes will help you feel stronger, wiser, and more powerful about your food choices. That can only improve your stress level!

My granddaughter Audrey grew up learning muscle-testing and energy-balancing. She has used the system you will learn in this book since she was five years old.

Audrey's Story

I'm working towards my bachelor's degree at Washington State University and I use the skills my grandparents taught me every day. I have used emotional clearing to help myself so much. I didn't gain those "freshman fifteen" pounds when I came to college, which I'm convinced is linked to the emotional stress that we are put under in leaving home for the first time. After leaving home for the first time, eating became a big comfort for me. My college is in a small town where there isn't much to do, so we eat out of boredom, too. I found that I had a lot of fear and worry and emptiness after leaving home. I have been able to clear my emotions when they come up and I also use muscle-testing to find my best foods. I have a small refrigerator in my dorm room in which I keep fresh vegetables for munching, and I cook some very tasty stir-frys in the community kitchen on my dorm floor.

If you feel like suppressed emotions are harming your ability to make good food choices, I can help with a simple technique to unblock those emotions. Go to TheFoodCodes.com.

CHAPTER 5
Muscle-Testing

The Holy Grail is within you – find your Inner Treasure.
– Jay Goodman

Now that you understand that food impacts your health and that it is intimately tied to your emotions and vitality, I bet you are eager to learn how to determine exactly what to eat. The Food Codes method is a deceptively simple way to discern what your body needs at any moment. People have a seemingly magical ability to know a truth from a lie. But it's not magic; it's an intuitive gift we all possess.

You can trust yourself to know what is right for you. You have all the answers you need right now to obtain optimal health and wellness. It's inside you, in what I call your "inner knower."

I once attended an energy-medicine seminar at which a well-known guest speaker spoke about internalized emotions. She asked for a volunteer from the audience to share something they were constantly struggling with. A woman went up on stage and talked about having gained weight since her divorce. The speaker then asked the woman a pointed question about her weight issue. The woman's answer to the question was

"I don't know." The speaker immediately blurted back to the woman, "Yes you do, and you know it in your knower!" The startled woman blinked in astonishment and then immediately spoke the answer.

Your inner knower is just another name for your subconscious mind, which is where you access your all-knowing intelligence. It's a data storage and retrieval system, but it's more complex than any computer. It's an unlimited memory bank of everything that has ever happened to you. It files sensations, impressions, and thoughts from all your senses. It never sleeps and constantly records information from your body and environment. It has the power to draw on forces of infinite intelligence. And you can access your inner knower at any time.

Muscle-testing is the technique you will use to access your subconscious mind. I teach this to my precious grandchildren, so you know it's safe. Anyone can do it, and it's fun.

Your body knows what foods it needs for health, what foods it needs to be trim and fit, and what foods might be causing you pain, inflammation, weight gain or loss, or symptoms of disease. The information is stored in your inner knower. Muscle-testing shows you how to access the information at home, at the grocery store, at a restaurant, and even in a buffet line on a cruise ship. You can use it silently and unobtrusively. No one will notice. They will only see that you are healthier and looking better than ever before.

Stop letting others tell you what to eat! Learn how to listen to your body and your own inner wisdom.

Every patient carries her or his own doctor inside.
– Albert Schweitzer

My husband, Bruce, taught me how to use muscle-testing. He used it with his chiropractic patients and taught many people how to use it in seminars. It was fascinating to watch Bruce use it to ask a patient what vertebra was out of alignment or what organ or gland was out of balance. Their body would immediately give the answer. We found that we could also ask what food was causing a bodily imbalance and what food would provide healing.

Ruthie's Story

Bruce's mother, Ruthie, was a lovely, small woman who was about seventy years old when she told me this story. She was demonstrating to my brother-in-law, Brigham, a young chiropractor, how to muscle-test. He was skeptical at first. Brigham had won the Mr. Northern California Bodybuilding competition, so he was a very strong guy.

Ruthie told him to hold one arm straight out to the side. She asked him to hold his arm steady and resist her pressure as he said, "My name is Brigham." She pressed down on his arm, and it was strong as a tree limb. She laughed and told me that you could have done chin-ups on his arm. Then she asked him to say, "My name is Bob," and he went weak as a willow and could not hold his arm up no matter how hard he tried. He was amazed and told her to do it again several times. Yet he was always weak and could not hold up his arm while saying something that was not true. He just kept saying, "I can't resist. How do you do that?"

Muscle-testing has been used by chiropractors, osteopathic doctors, neurologists, physical therapists, and other professionals for over forty years. When I was introduced to it, it worked right away and I got very strong answers. I would ask Bruce to test things for me. For instance, I would be making lunch and pull out a half-full jar of mayonnaise from the fridge, wonder if it was still good, and ask him, "Honey, will you test this for me to see if it's still good?" That worked fabulously, except that "Honey" was not always available when I wanted something tested, so I had to learn muscle-testing myself.

The Power of Your Subconscious Mind

Your subconscious mind, sometimes called the unconscious brain or the body-mind, holds and is continuously recording your existence. It's in a state of "record on" day and night, recording every bit of information in your environment and every thought and emotion. Your conscious mind can process only a tiny fraction of the information that the subconscious mind processes per second. The subconscious mind knows which stresses have taken your body to an energetically imbalanced state, as well as what your body needs to return to a state of balance and harmony.

The conscious mind is not usually aware of all the underlying stressors causing the body to be out of balance or unhealthy. We think we need to eat more broccoli, take vitamins, drink green smoothies, or avoid carbohydrates because that is what we hear in the media. However, each person is unique and has specific nutritional needs that can vary with the seasons, the amount of stress they are experiencing, and, for a woman, the phase of her menstrual cycle. Your subconscious mind knows all this information and can communicate it to you easily!

You can access the information in your subconscious mind by using muscle-testing, which a form of biofeedback. It is also called manual muscle testing (MMT), and kinesiology by some. *Biofeedback* is information received from the body in response to a question or internal stimulus like a thought. It is usually performed using a device connected to the body by wires. A lie detector test works in the same way. Through muscle-testing the human body gives a yes or no answer in reaction to a question or even a thought. This is a way to receive answers held deeply in the subconscious mind, and it will not lie; it always tells the truth.

Muscle-testing is much like traditional biofeedback, only it's wireless. Haven't we all gone wireless these days? You can use it anywhere and anytime.

As tools, our hands are the most sensitive, fine-tuned instruments available...this instrument we call the hand is hooked up to the most marvelous computer ever created. It is the examiner's very own personal computer.
– Florence P. Kendall

This most marvelous computer that Florence P. Kendall speaks of is, of course, your subconscious mind, and it's a gift that is always available to help you and give you the information you seek.

There are several different techniques you can use to muscle-test. I use different methods in different situations. I suggest that you try out the different methods described below to determine your favorite, or the one that is easiest for you to use at first. Once you get comfortable with that method you can practice the others to explore their feasibility for you.

Eight Tips for Muscle-Testing Success

You can do this!

1. Find one method that feels and works best for you, practice it until you feel comfortable with it, then try the others.

2. Before beginning, relax and take a few deep breaths, clearing any anticipation of a particular outcome.

3. Ask simple yes or no questions.

4. Use the minimum of pressure. This is a gentle technique.

5. Establish a baseline by asking an easy question.

6. *Intend* that you will receive a strong yes or a weak no. (More about this below.)

7. Get permission before testing others. A parent or guardian can give permission for a child under eighteen years of age.

8. Be patient and practice to progress! You are training your mind and muscles to respond just as an athlete in a training program does.

For video demos of these testing methods, visit TheFoodCodes.com.

The Sway Method

This is the best one to start with because it's simple and the results are very clear. Practice it at home until you feel confident. I love the sway test because almost anyone can do it immediately. Many professionals use this as their primary testing method.

Stand comfortably straight yet relaxed. It is normal for your body to move a little while you are standing. Your eyes can be

Muscle-Testing

open or closed, but keep them open if it helps you keep your balance. It can also be done while sitting in a chair. Sit forward on the chair so you have room to sway.

Your inner knower naturally leans toward positivity and is drawn to the truth. Negativity and lies are quite the opposite; you steer away from negativity and push backward from a lie. This is the biofeedback reaction I described earlier.

1. Pick a loving thought. Imagine a newborn baby; a soft, cuddly puppy; or a warm, sweet kiss. Embrace that thought. Sink into it. Feel how yummy it is.
2. Your body sways forward.
3. This is your body saying yes.

Now switch your thinking:

1. Bring in a negative thought – something disgusting or sad. Hold that thought. Sink deeper as the thought gets stronger.
2. Your body sways backward.
3. This is your body saying no.

That yes and no are your baseline – one yes answer and one no answer. Always establish your baseline. It shows that you are "testable" and able to connect to your subconscious mind, your inner knower.

If at any time you feel you are not getting a correct answer, stop; reestablish your baseline by asking for a firm yes and a weak no; then ask the question again. (See tips below for switching your thinking if you have trouble doing this.) The following instructions walk you through establishing your baseline for each method.

The Food Codes: Intuitive Eating for Every Body

Muscle-Testing with a Partner

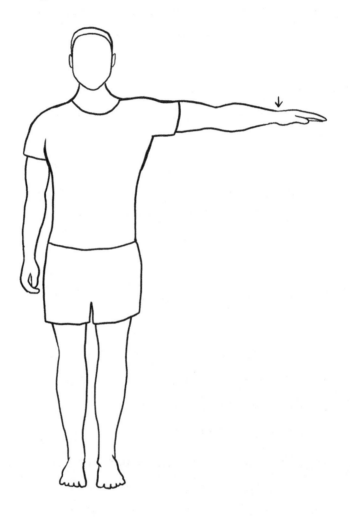

Chose a partner who is willing to be tested and does not have arm or shoulder problems. They don't need to know a thing about muscle-testing.

1. Face your partner and have them hold their arm out to the side, parallel to the floor. Place your fingers just above the wrist bump of their arm. Place your other hand lightly on their other shoulder for stability.

2. Be gentle. Tell your partner to resist you gently, and with your hand that is on their wrist slowly press down. Use the least amount of pressure that is needed to feel their resistance – the yes answer – and stop pressing.

3. With your partner's arm out to the side again, have them say their name: "My name is _____ ." Gently and slowly press down on their arm until you feel it stop or lock, then stop pressing. Don't let their arm bounce; just press and stop when you feel their arm lock into a stop. This can feel strong or subtle depending on the individual. This is a yes. Release the position.

4. With your partner's arm out to the side again, have them say, "My name is _____," using any name that is not theirs. Press down gently on their arm. Their arm will be weak or drop all the way down; you will not feel the lock. Immediately stop pressing; don't throw their arm downward.

Have fun with this and switch back and forth. You be the subject next and have them test you.

The Food Codes: Intuitive Eating for Every Body

The Arm Self-Test Method

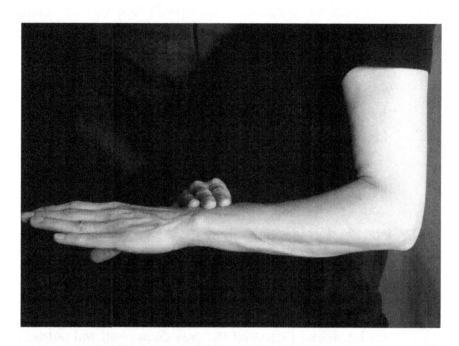

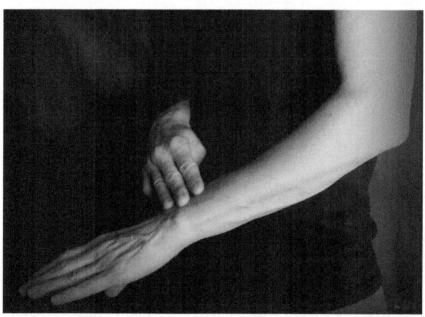

1. Hold either arm to your side and bend it forward at the elbow to form a right angle. You might find that one arm works better than the other at first – probably your nondominant arm.
2. Using your other hand, place two or three fingers just above the wrist bump of your arm.
3. Say, "Show me a yes," and slowly push downward until you feel resistance, then stop. This is your yes.
4. Say, "Show me a no," and slowly push downward. Your arm will drop without much resistance. This is your no.

The Food Codes: Intuitive Eating for Every Body

The Interlocking Ring Method

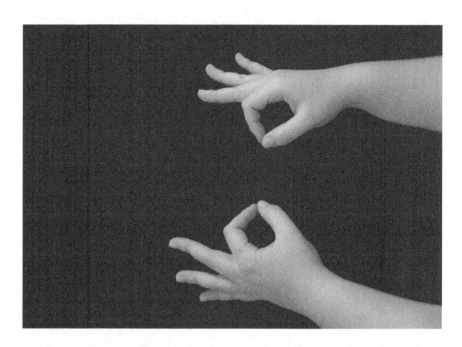

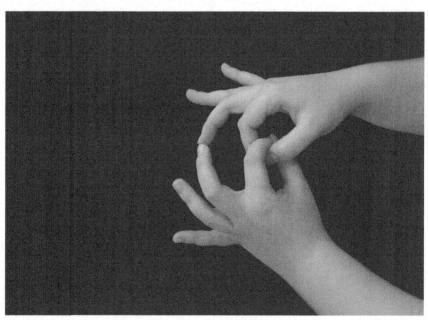

Muscle-Testing

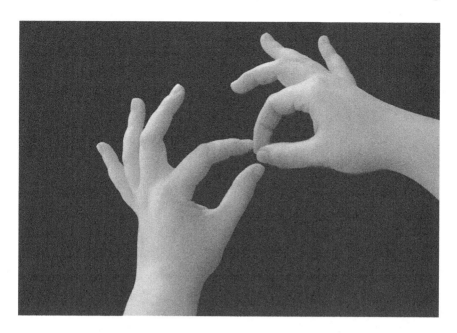

1. Make "finger rings," or "okay" signs, with both hands by placing your thumbs and index fingers together, with your other fingers relaxed yet held up.

2. Open the finger and thumb of one hand and link your hands together with two interlocking rings.

3. Say, "Show me a yes," and slowly try to pull your finger rings apart. Stop pulling when you feel resistance. Your fingers will feel almost like they are sticking together. This is your yes. This is a gentle action. Don't yank or pull with force.

4. Open your fingers and relax them, then interlock your finger rings again.

5. Say, "Show me a no," and slowly try to pull your finger rings apart. There should be no resistance as the fingers slide easily apart. The fingers on one hand might stay together while the fingers on the other hand release. This is your no.

The Food Codes: Intuitive Eating for Every Body

The Hole and Finger Method

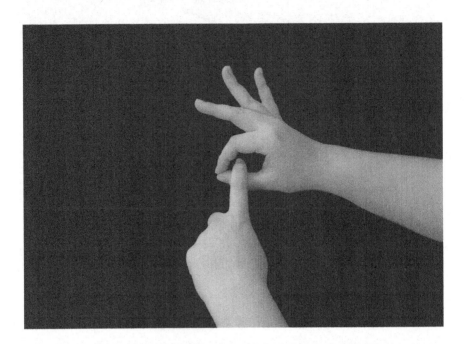

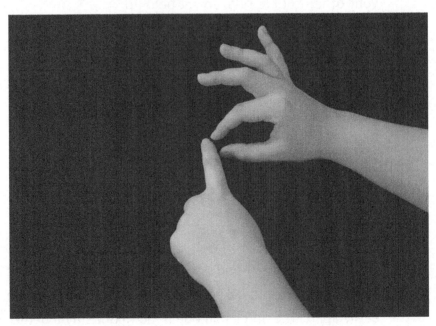

1. Make a finger ring with your nondominant hand. (The rest of the instructions assume you are right-handed and have made the ring with your left hand.)

2. Insert your right index finger into the finger ring and say, "Show me a yes," and slowly try to pull your finger through the ring, breaking the connection. Stop when you feel resistance. The ring will feel like it is stuck together. This is your yes. Relax your hands.

3. Form the finger ring again, insert the other index finger, say, "Show me a no," and slowly pull your finger through the ring. It will easily slide through. This is your no.

The Food Codes: Intuitive Eating for Every Body

The Finger-Ring Push-Apart Method

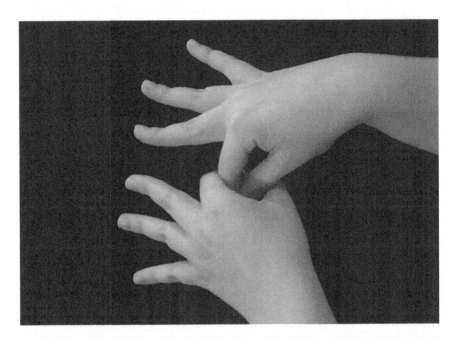

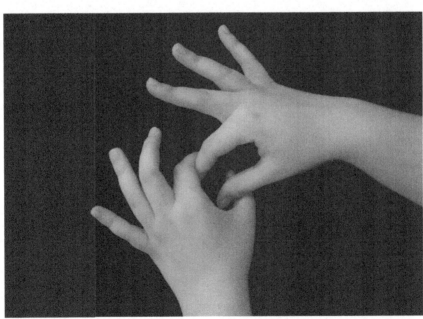

1. Make a finger ring with your nondominant hand. (The rest of the instructions assume you are right-handed and have made the ring with your left hand.)

2. With your right hand, make the shape of a bird's beak with your thumb and index finger.

3. Insert the beak into the finger ring (from above or below, it makes no difference).

4. Say, "Show me a yes," and slowly try to push the finger ring apart with the beak fingers. Stop pushing when you feel resistance. Your finger ring will feel almost like your index finger is stuck to your thumb. This is your yes. Be gentle. Don't force it. Relax your hands.

5. Start over and say, "Show me a no," and slowly try to push your finger ring apart. You should have no resistance and the finger ring opens easily. This is your no.

The Index Finger Method

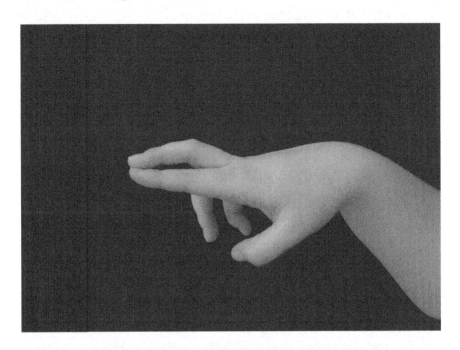

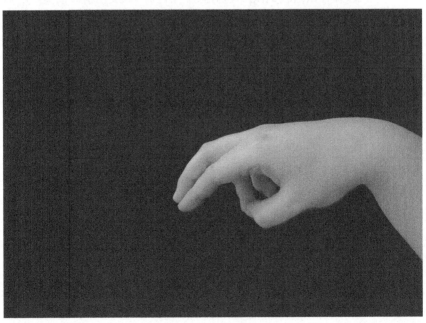

I love this method because it can be done very discretely in a restaurant when you are using it to determine what foods your body requires.

1. Hold either index finger out and cross your middle finger on top of it.
2. Say, "Show me a yes," and slowly push down on your index finger. Stop when you feel resistance. Relax your hands.
3. Say, "Show me a no," and slowly push down on your finger. There will be no resistance.

You can try other finger combinations to see if any work better than the middle finger over the index finger. I have seen this method used with any finger as the testing finger.

Dowsing, Pendulums

A dowsing device, pendulum, can also be used to test for answers. A pendulum is a weight suspended from a cord, chain, or string that swings freely to indicate a yes or no answer. There are also a variety of dowsing devices available that indicate a yes or no.

Practice, Practice, Practice

I didn't master muscle-testing immediately. I had to practice – a lot. Now it feels like second nature. If you have to work to get good results, take heart and know that it just takes practice.

Practice puts brains in your muscles.
– Samuel Snead

After practicing your baseline yeses and nos, ask questions to which you know the answers as you practice through the day to replicate your baseline results. Ask precise yes or no questions, not complex ones. You are *training* your muscles to give you the answers you *tell* yourself are correct. While you're practicing it's perfectly okay to make your muscles resist for a yes and go weak for a no. For example, you walk into your kitchen and notice an apple on the counter:

1. Say, "This is an apple," then tell yourself, "Give me a strong yes."
2. Next you say, "This is an orange," then tell yourself, "Give me a weak no."
3. You can also *ask*, "Is this an apple?" and tell yourself, "Give me a strong yes"; and ask, "Is this an orange?" and tell yourself, "Give me a weak no."

Examples of precise yes or no questions:

- Do I have dog?
- Am I a female?
- Am I married?
- Do I have a sister?
- Is my birthday in December?

Don't ask complex questions:

- Why do I love country music?
- How do I drive to Boston?
- When will I get a promotion?
- What is my spouse thinking about?
- Should I eat spinach cooked or fresh?

Using the spinach example, you can first ask, "Is spinach a good food for me at this time?" If the answer is yes, you can ask, "Is it okay to eat fresh spinach?" and you can ask, "Is it better to eat cooked spinach?"

What NOT to Use Muscle-Testing For

- Predicting the future.
- Playing the lottery or gambling.
- Situations in which you are emotionally involved.
- Making big life-changing decisions. These are best decided through meditation and prayer.

Mary's Story

Mary called me very frustrated and said she just could not do the muscle-testing. I calmly asked which method she was trying to use, and she talked on and on about her frustrations trying to use that one particular method. When I asked if she had tried any of the other methods, she said, "Oh yes. I don't have any problem using other methods." Then she added loudly, "But this is the one I want to use!" I counseled her to be patient, that probably in time she would master it, and for now to use one of the other methods that was comfortable for her.

How to Correct Switching

What I call "switching" is when you get wrong answers while perfecting your muscle-testing. You might also get all nos or all yeses. Here are some ways to correct either of these:

1. Tap or slap each shoulder several times with your opposite hand.

2. In the following steps you use your *governing meridian* – a primary acupuncture meridian that transmits energy from your tailbone up and over your head, ending at your upper lip – to focus your body. Chinese medicine tells us that this meridian "governs" the other meridians flowing through the body.

    a. Swipe the top of your head from front to back with your hand as you think or say aloud, "My yes is a strong answer," three or four times.

    b. Retest your yes using the muscle-testing method of your choice.

    c. Take a nice deep breath and relax for moment.

    d. Swipe the top of your head from front to back with your hand as you think or say aloud, "My no is a weak answer," three or four times.

    e. Retest your no using the muscle-testing method of your choice.

3. Drink a tall glass of water. Hydration is very important in conducting electricity through your body, which facilitates the travel of energy through your body.

4. Stretch your neck side to side, shoulder to shoulder, and up and down may help to realign your muscles and vertebrae. Misalignment of the neck can affect energy flow.

Our intention is everything. Nothing on this planet happens without it. Not one single thing has ever been accomplished without intention.
– Jim Carrey

Set an Intention for Better Muscle-Testing

Setting an intention with the help of the method I teach you next, can help you manifest quicker and easier muscle-testing results. This can help if you are a little unsure of yourself.

It is simple to set an intention that instantly fills your entire body using the radiant energy of your hands, and your governing meridian. Your hands emit energy naturally. (You might have heard the term *healing hands* or know something about *healing touch*.)

1. Set your intention for your yes by swiping the top of your head from front to back with your hand while thinking or saying out loud, "My yes is a strong, resistant answer."

2. Set your intention for your no by swiping the top of your head from front to back with your hand, while thinking or saying out loud, "My no is a weak answer."

This works for all methods of muscle-testing. You can also use a magnet to set an intention, which is explained in the following section.

Using a Magnet to Balance Energy

Magnets are very effective in restoring balance to the body. Ancient Egyptians, Romans, Greeks, and Chinese used magnets in this way, and they are used today in meditation practices and to relieve pain. Bruce and his brother, Bradley, use special magnetic devises to help clear and balance their patients.

Magnets have an energy field that can be physically measured. Even a simple refrigerator magnet has an energy field. If you put a magnet close to a credit card, it will erase the magnetic information on the card.

Your fingers and palm emit an energy field just as a magnet does. In the following balancing exercise, you can use just your hand instead of a magnet.

Energy-Balancing Exercise: Setting an Intention

Swipe the top of your head from front to back with a magnet, the palm of your hand, or your fingertips while saying or thinking, "Come into balance," three or four times, then take a nice deep breath.

I have used this swiping method as described for twenty-plus years. It works amazingly well. Bruce eventually moved away from manually adjusting his patients' bones and instead uses this swiping method with a magnet, rolling the magnet down the entire governing meridian of the patient's back to balance and realign.

The Muscle-Testing Bonus

Muscle-testing sharpens your intuition and your ability to immediately access your inner knower – that all-knowing subconscious mind of yours. As you practice and use muscle-testing, you will find that your answers seem to pop into your mind, or you might "feel" the answer or just know the answer. When this happens it might make you doubt the muscle-testing technique because you think you must be influencing your answers. ...And you are influencing your answers! When you muscle-test the answer pops up instantly from your subconscious. You feel or know the answer a split second before it manifests in your body. This is in essence why muscle-testing works, and this sharpening of your intuition is the bonus! Go to TheFoodCodes.com for tips on muscle-testing.

Christine suffered with colon cancer and had surgery to remove the affected area. "What can I eat?" was her biggest worry. She had digestion and liver problems, severe bowel pain, and flatulence, and was exhausted for many years.

Christine's Story

I had no problems using the food plan. It is very clear even though I live in another country and we don't have the same terms.

Using the Food Codes plan, I realized that my body knows exactly what is appropriate. Most of the foods I was eating before I got the food plan were in conformity with the food plan. That gave me great self-confidence with my own intuition.

Then there were foods I would really like to eat but didn't allow myself to eat because of old beliefs like "these are not good for you because they have too much protein." When the Food Codes plan showed me that these foods were also very good for me I could let go of these old and stuck beliefs and enjoy these foods, too.

With the Food Codes plan, I also knew exactly what wasn't good for me, for example coffee. Some health experts tell you now to drink coffee for health. I felt it was bad for my health but I had been drinking it anyway. The food plan showed me that my feeling was right; coffee is not good for me. And with that I again gained self-confidence in my inner knowingness.

In short terms, the benefit for me from the Food Codes plan was to "trust in self" and "let go of old stuck beliefs in relation to food."

The two most significant improvements I noticed from using the food plan were more energy after eating – feeling energized and not tired, and less flatulence and better digestion.

What I learned from using the Food Codes is that I'm able to listen to my body. My body or my inner knowingness knows exactly what is good for me. For me it is important to listen to myself and to gain more self-confidence.

Using the Food Codes for over a year has given me a good feeling that I can support my health. Eating according to the food plan gives me energy. I'm energized after eating and I do not have flatulence. For me the food plan is something that gives me joy, it is not a "must." It gives me trust and self-confidence every time when my body asks for a special food and I realize that this food is exactly in harmony with my food plan. With that I learned to listen to my body. I learned to trust my body. It has its own intelligence and knows exactly what is needed. The Food Codes plan is a very precious support, and I think unique, because it refers to energy; it shows me which food is the most energizing food for me right now.

I thank you from my heart for your precious work. This is a true gift.

The Food Codes System

In this part of *The Food Codes* you'll refer to the Food Codes Food List of foods, beverages, and condiments. Using the muscle-testing techniques you learned in the previous chapter, you'll go through each list and test whether or not the food is beneficial for you. I suggest you give each food a numerical ranking from 0 to 10 and write down the number.

Go to TheFoodCodes.com/lists and download and print the free PDF of the Food Codes Food List so you can write on it. Keep a blank original for copying when you need to update your Food Codes.

CHAPTER 6
Unlocking Your Food Codes

Tell me what you eat, and I will tell you what you are.
– Jean Anthelme Brillat-Savarin

The newest BIG-DEAL diet discovery is "Not all foods work for all people!" What an astounding discovery! Add some sarcasm when you read that, because I discovered this more than two decades ago. These new diets tell you to start the diet using their general list of foods and see how it works for you. If this doesn't work start deleting foods one at a time to see what happens. When you find, through trial and error, *over several weeks,* what foods are good for you, eat those foods until you get the desired result. Wonderful! The final step is to add foods that you deleted back into your diet one at a time to see if they are still bad for you. I'm not sure how many weeks this could take, and I'm not sure how many people would persevere on this diet. I know I wouldn't want to.

Muscle-testing to find your best foods works in mere seconds. You can discover in minutes all the foods that are good for you and bad for you and be on your way to your local market with a grocery list. Muscle-testing works for rating foods because each food has a unique frequency that communicates to your inner knower, whether or not you should eat it to help balance and enhance your body's energy. You will test what foods you should eat to nourish your body, release weight, or enhance your workout program.

Frequencies of foods, herbs, and essential oils can be tested with devices that use the Hertz scale. But just because a food or herb has a very high frequency rating on the Hertz scale, doesn't mean that it's the best for you at any given time. The Food Codes method shows you what foods you need right now, to bring balance to your body and help raise your vibrational energy.

Amy's Story

Hi Lana! I am so appreciative of all the amazing work you have done with me this year with the Body Code and Emotion Code. For the past eight years I have been practicing and receiving myofascial release – which has been very effective in releasing many of the underlying causes of much pain and trauma. The Body Code and Emotion Code are quite surprising in how specific the information obtained is and the ease of releasing. My sessions with you have helped me make many monumental changes in my physical as well as emotional health in a short period of four months.

Food is a particular issue that I have struggled with my whole life. I have had allergies and food sensitivities since I was a young child. I have tried so many different approaches, elimination diets, specialized diets, and I am in a constant state of experimentation as to what foods I can eat and feel healthy.

No one seemed to have a comprehensive idea as to what I should eat.

Most recently I was starting to have bloating issues – spontaneously after eating something my belly would protrude out of nowhere. My naturopath suggested that I had small intestine bacterial overgrowth (SIBO), and I proceeded with a simple carbohydrate diet. I had a suspicion that it had something to do with salt, but no one could confirm that was likely, so I ignored it. Improvements were made with the SIBO diet, but I did not feel like I was really on track. I continued to experiment with food.

As soon as I received my food list from you – foods my body REALLY likes and REALLY doesn't like, I printed up the list and followed it fairly purely. I was not surprised to find salt and sea salt on the list of foods my body does not like – this would be the first time I tried eliminating it from my diet. I quickly figured out that I could not eat anything packaged from a store or eat out at a restaurant unless I could do a special order. This requires me to make everything from scratch at home. Now I KNOW that my body is very sensitive to salt and sea salt. I have not had problems with the Himalayan pink salt, which showed up as a desirable food. What a difference!

There were other foods I was not aware that my body did not like – kale? Pea protein? Stevia? Rice pasta? Rice flour? I was eating a lot of these. I have been gluten sensitive for many years and usually avoid it, missing bread often. This food list included sourdough bread as a food my body REALLY likes! Yes, I have now tested it many times and find it has a completely different response in my body – no gluten symptoms at all. "WE" like sourdough bread! I can now eat a sandwich again!

Dairy products are not on my desirable list, which I suspected. But lo-and-behold, one kind of cheese was there Dubliner! I had not tried it before, but it does agree with my body – it is a real treat with no aftereffects. How would I ever figure that out on my own?

I always loved spinach in my smoothies. I was told that fresh spinach can deplete or block calcium from your body, yet fresh spinach tested high for me and so I returned to using it rather than kale.

I asked you to test specific supplements that I was taking – whole-food supplements that were high quality and also high cost. My intuition had been questioning them. You found they did not test high for me at this time and I have since stopped taking them and feel better, also saving me significant money!

I found myself to be highly sensitive to eggs after doing a juice fast and becoming violently ill after introducing eggs back into my diet. I have avoided eating eggs for several years and have really missed them. Despite this, eggs tested high for me on the food list as desirable. You did some clearing for me to find out why my body was responding to the eggs this way. I had an intolerance to "one bad egg from a specific time" and that was cleared. I can now eat eggs – some of the time. The food list also confirmed many discoveries that I had made about sensitivities to dairy, gluten, sugar, and corn.

I am now eating according to what my BODY wants to eat and I feel so much better. This is what I have been striving for all along and I feel so relieved to have a method to communicate with my body and find out exactly what it wants and needs.

Mentally, I feel more confident about this method of food testing because it is so specific to just ME and my unique physical, chemical, emotional self! It is confirmed to me in many ways. I am excited to see how it may change over time periods with retesting to meet ongoing needs.

Thank you so much for your wonderful work. It is as if you read my mind (which you probably did!) with the timing of the food list – it saved me from seeking out yet another experiment of figuring out foods for myself.

Ahhh, love and hugs!

The Food Codes Testing Methods

We each have our own style of learning. If you love to analyze and research, and you always want more details, I suggest using Method 1 below to test foods. You will love the precise, detailed results from this method.

If you like to jump in, move fast, and just zoom to the finish line to get it done, Method 2 is for you. That said, I suggest you use Method 1 the first few times you test your Food Codes plan. Your eyes will be opened to a new understanding of your amazing body and its ever-changing nutritional needs. I guarantee doing this will lead you to a deeper, more intimate and meaningful relationship with your divine friend, food.

The foods that test very low for you right now could easily test better for you at another time. The same applies to foods that test high for you now; they could change to lower values at a future date. This should teach you to *stop judging food* and appreciate its life-sustaining qualities.

Start here: Download a free copy of the Food Codes Food List at TheFoodCodes.com/lists.

Method 1
Muscle-Test Using a Scale of 0 to 10

Using muscle-testing, ask how healthy each item on the Food Codes Food List is for you at this time and rate each one on a scale of 0 to 10, with 0 being low and 10 being high.

Example: Ask, "On a scale of 0 to 10, how good is this food for me at this time? Is it a 0? 1? 2?" (and so on).

After you finish testing your list, ask, "How long is this Food Codes plan good for? Is it days? Weeks? Months?"

Begin by eating only foods that test 8, 9, or 10, adding a few that test 5, 6, and 7 as needed. Avoiding foods that test lower than 5 will help you feel better. These could be the foods that drain your energy.

Method 2
Muscle-Test Using Xs and 0s

After you learn the value of rating foods by using Method 1, try Method 2, the quickie method, in which you don't have to ask about each rate. Rather than rating foods from 0 to 10, mark an X on the best foods and a 0 (zero) on the foods to avoid.

Move through the Food Codes Food List asking or thinking this question: "What are my best foods at this time?" Mark an X beside each food that tests "best" for you. These will be foods that would rate an 8, 9, or 10 using Method 1.

Next ask, "What foods should I avoid at this time?" Mark a 0 by these foods. These will be foods that would rate from 0 to 4 using Method 1.

Foods that would rate 5, 6, or 7 will be left without a rating. You end up with a list you can glance through quickly to see what foods are your best and what foods to avoid. You can eat those without a rating on occasion.

Now ask, "How long is this Food Codes plan good for? Days? Weeks? Months?"

Retest foods whenever you want to, using the answers to the time-frame question as a guide. If you are under a lot of stress, have the flu, or are traveling, you can test to see what you need to eat in that moment to support your health.

Brenda's Story

Brenda had tummy aches constantly as a child, and her parents took her to one doctor after another. They could find nothing wrong with her stomach, and more than one physician told her parents she was just trying to get attention. She would have bouts of diarrhea, gas, and bulging tummy. Her skin would break out in rashes that itched like crazy.

She was eventually told that she had many food allergies. She became very thin and depressed in high school and her friends whispered that she was anorexic. Growing up was hard for Brenda. Seeking out help from professionals, she received conflicting advice about the cause of her problem, what to eat, and what not to eat, and was prescribed various medications. Brenda heard me speak about my food plan on a talk show and immediately contacted me for help.

On the advice of a health food expert, she had been juicing vegetables and eating raw foods for almost two years, wondering when this method of eating was going to pay off. Her husband complained that there was nothing but raw carrots and celery in the fridge.

In testing for Brenda's first Food Codes plan we found that she needed mostly cooked food and only an occasional raw salad for the first three months. She needed to cook or steam all her vegetables and she needed meat proteins, rich bone broth, and a lot of fats. Organic beef, liver, and wild game; full-fat yogurt and butter; and flax oil and olive oil tested as some of her top foods.

This was Brenda's comment about her first Food Codes plan: "Thank you, Lana. This Food Codes plan sure feels right. There are some surprising things in this listing that no other food plan has ever recognized, but I know they are right. I should have trusted my intuition a long time ago, even though it went against so-called experts' advice. I'm excited about this!"

Brenda learned to test her foods to discover her best foods. She lost her gaunt, skinny, unhealthy appearance and her skin recovered from the years of scaly, itchy rashes. She gained weight and found some lovely curves to her body. She sent me a wonderful recipe that she created for homemade sausage which she makes from her husband's wild game. And he loves her new curves!

After Testing

By concentrating on your highest-ranking foods you'll effortlessly release weight if your body needs to reduce, or gain weight, if that's what you need. Your subconscious mind knows exactly what you need to eat and drink to give you optimal health.

You'll have created your own personal Food Codes plan! Imagine how easy your life will be – no more counting calories, guilt about eating the wrong thing, or confusion about the latest fad diet.

You can take the Food Codes testing to another level by doing the exercise below to create more specific lists; for example, a list of foods to provide you with more energy at work. You can ask what foods your child needs right now to balance their body and brain or to boost their energy for final exams.

Be sure to create your general Food Codes plan first as a baseline, even though it might be very similar to a plan that your body chooses for a specific issue like a health problem or weight loss. Your inner knower knows what you need.

Muscle-Testing Exercise for Specific Needs

Ask, "Do I need a specific Food Codes plan?" Even if the answer is no, move on to testing foods for your goal. If the answer is yes, ask if it is one of the plans listed below. If so, then use the list below to test and see which specific plan your body requires. If the answer is no, move on to testing foods for your goal. Check your results by asking, "Is this best for me now?" You might want to target weight loss when what you really need right now is to simply balance your body.

Specific Food Codes Plans

- Balance my body
- Weight loss
- A certain health condition
- Athletic training
- Beauty – skin, hair, etc.
- Hydration

- Brain and memory
- Increased energy
- Cleanse or detoxification
- Juicing

Trust Your Subconscious

Your results will often surprise you. You might find out that your body wants more of a food that you've been taught was unhealthy, like butter. Or you might be encouraged to eat something you have not cared for in the past, like beets or turnips. Experiment and trust your results. Try the foods for a few days and see how you feel. You could feel an increase in energy or mental clarity or sleep better.

Once you become confident in your ability to test foods, you can walk into the grocery store and test to see which apples are best for you. You can test to see if your body craves organic strawberries or regular ones. You can determine which vitamins and supplements your body requires. You can test everything that goes into your body, even how many glasses of water you should drink.

You can test to see whether your body wants a food cooked or raw. Some people are unable to eat raw broccoli because it has a negative impact on their thyroid, while cooked broccoli is just fine for them. It is as easy as asking, "Should I eat my green beans raw?" and "Should I eat my green beans cooked?"

Kurt's Story

The Food Codes are very easy to read and use. I focused on not eating the foods that tested "not good" for me and I tried to eat more of the foods that tested "very good" for me.

The two most significant improvements I noticed were I got more energy, and the flatulence and the expanded stomach released and disappeared almost completely after three or four weeks.

To be honest, I know more or less what is not good for me, but to use the healing Food Codes plan information in black and white is a stronger instruction and guidance, and it is easy for me to follow.

Testing Pets and Animals

We adore our pets and want them to be happy. So we don't want what we lovingly feed our pets to be bad for them. Many of us have the same confusion about what to feed our pets that we have about what to feed ourselves! "How do I know what foods are best for my cat?" "Is it okay to feed my dog, people food?" "What bird seed is best for Polly?" "My vet tells me one thing and experts say something totally different. Who can I trust?"

Our fur babies need their Food Codes tested, too. It works the same for all animals, large or small, as it does for humans. Just like a human, an animal has different food requirements at different times and at different stages of life. Along with good food they might need supplemental nutrition, and they also require good water, air, and sunshine for their best health.

One of my clients, a Holland lop bunny rabbit named Sissy, had an allergy to carrots. We tested that apples were instead one of her best foods. Another client, Elvis, a long-haired guinea pig with an Elvis Presley poof of hair, also had a problem eating carrots. Lettuce was at the top of his Food Codes plan.

Roxy, my daughter's family boxer dog, had lost patches of hair on her back. The veterinarian checked her and said she was in good health, and that the hair loss was fairly common for older boxers. We tested Roxy's Food Codes and found that she needed to eat cooked chicken meat, take a supplement for her thyroid gland, and switch to another type of dog food. Her hair loss improved.

Testing your animals' Food Codes is easy, takes the guesswork out of feeding them, and saves money on food and supplements. You can test a horse in a pasture or a dog on your lap. You don't have to hold or touch them. You set an intention that you are testing yourself for the animal. Be sure to get the owner's permission to test an animal that is not your own.

Muscle-Testing Method for Animals

1. Use the muscle-testing method that works best for you while touching, holding, or simply thinking about the animal.

2. You can use another person, ideally the animal's owner, as a surrogate to test an animal, following the instructions for muscle-testing with a partner in Chapter 5. Have your partner connect with the animal by touching, holding, or simply thinking of it. Your partner becomes the conduit through which the answers flow.

3. Establish baseline yes and no answers.

4. You can ask specific questions with yes or no answers, like "Is XYZ brand of dog food best for Fido at this time?" or value questions like "On a scale of 0 to 10, how good is XYZ dog food for Fido? 0? 1? 2? [etc.]."

5. You can also use the Food Codes Food List to find foods that might test best for Fido.

6. When you finish testing, disconnect from the animal by saying, "My name is [your name]" a few times until you receive a yes. Have your partner do the same if you're using a partner.

7. Check with the animal's veterinarian or health care provider before changing foods, supplements, or exercise routines. A food that should *not* be fed to your animal might test as a good food. Investigate a little further to see what nutrients that food contains that the animal might need, but don't feed that food. Check with the animal's veterinarian or health care provider if you have further questions.

Topics to Test for Animals
- What are the best foods for them?
- What foods should they avoid?
- What is the best brand of food for them?
- Is canned food better for them?
- Is dry food better for them?
- What supplements, vitamins, and minerals do they need?
- Is tap water okay for them?
- Is purified water better for them?
- Are raw foods better for them?
- Are cooked foods better for them?

CHAPTER 7

Living Well with Your Food Codes Plan

We are indeed much more than what we eat, but what we eat can nevertheless help us to be much more than what we are.
– Adele Davis

Now that you have completed testing for your personal Food Codes, you can glean more information about your health and your needs by examining the Food Codes Food List for some interesting insights. If you see dairy products with very low ratings, for example, they could be the reason you have gas and bloating.

You can test high for a food you are allergic to if it contains a nutrient your body needs. If you are allergic to any food that tests high for you, please use good sense and avoid that food.

Unlike most diets, on this food plan you can eat whatever you want to whenever you want to. That alone can make you feel more at ease. But if you want to *reach your ideal weight and increase the balance of energy in your body*, it's as simple as 1, 2, 3:

1. Eat the foods that have the highest ratings.

2. Eat only when you are hungry.

3. Stop eating when you are full.

1. Eat the foods that have the highest ratings.

Eat them alone or combine them with other foods rated high in recipes for soups, stews, and casseroles. You can add a lower-rated food to a recipe if it will add flavor or enhance the dish. For example, if you're making a meatloaf that calls for chopped onion, but onion is a three on your plan, add just a little onion for flavor and texture if it would enhance your joy in eating the meatloaf. But leave the food out if it is a 0, 1, or 2; or if it is a food you are allergic to.

2. Eat only when you are hungry.

Babies and small children refuse food when they're not hungry. Somewhere along the way many of us lost the ability to recognize what it feels like when we're full. We schedule breakfast, lunch, and dinner at certain times and eat at those times because that is what we are trained to do. We eat out of habit at break time at work, or when we see a brownie sitting on the counter. Sometimes we think we are hungry when we are actually thirsty. And sometimes emotions pop up that send us to the refrigerator when we're not hungry.

Learn to feel hunger inside before eating. This takes practice and remembering innate instincts. Practice asking yourself, "On a scale of 0 to 10 how hungry am I? 0? 1? 2? [etc.]" If you don't feel hungry but you want to be able to join your family or colleagues for the next scheduled meal, enjoy eating a little something, yet not a full meal. Otherwise simply enjoy the company and just wait to eat until you actually feel hungry.

3. Stop eating when you are full.

With jumbo-sized restaurant portions, all-you-can-eat buffets, and a culture that encourages us to stuff ourselves full of food, many of us no longer recognize the feeling of fullness in our stomachs because we've been ignoring that sensation for so long. Babies know how to do this instinctively. When you try to get a little one to eat more than she wants, she'll turn her head, spit food out, or throw her bowl to the floor. (But I'm not encouraging you to do that!)

Many of us were trained to clean our plates when we were kids. It takes some time and practice to reconnect to the sensation of being full, but you can test for that as well. I did an experiment recently with a cup of chicken noodle soup. As I ate it, I paid attention to the taste and how good it felt in my mouth. When there was just a tiny bit left in the cup, I felt a "slam" in my energy field that told me what I needed to know. I looked down into my cup and thought, "Well, there're just a couple of sips left. I could just finish this instead of wasting it." I heard my mother telling me about the starving children. But I decided to honor my body and pour the rest of the soup in the disposer. It felt really good, almost liberating.

Muscle-Testing for Hunger

Use muscle-testing to confirm your intuition regarding the sensations of hunger and fullness. Honor your body by not feeding it when it does not need food. If you only eat when you're hungry, it lifts from your body the burden of eating to satisfy a schedule. It helps you retain your natural energy level. It also helps you enjoy your food more. Even a piece of dry, crusty bread can taste delicious when you are really hungry; food is not only more satisfying but is more beneficial to your body.

So before you eat, ask yourself, "Am I hungry? Am I really hungry to eat now?" Get a gauge on that by using your intuition and muscle-testing. I ask myself, "How hungry am I right now, on a scale of 0 to 10? 0? 1? 2? [etc.]" If I am at least a 6 on the hunger scale, I'll eat.

As you are eating, muscle-test periodically by asking, "Am I full?" Then gage how full you are. You might be surprised by how quickly you actually fill up. I have found that if I stop eating when I am at a 6, I feel good and satisfied as I finish my meal. Keep in mind that it takes a bit of time for the feeling of satiety to register in your brain. Eating slowly allows you to notice this as it happens. If you find yourself eating to the fullness of a 9 or 10, you may feel stuffed, bloated, and uncomfortable after eating. You know… that feeling of "Oh, I may never eat again!"

Most of my clients tell me that they feel better when they stop eating at a fullness level of 5 or 6. Experiment by stopping at 5, 6, 7, and 8 at different meals to find out what level is best for you, based on how you feel a little while after eating.

Use this strategy like a training exercise for getting healthy, fit, and trim. You will relearn the feelings of hunger and fullness that you instinctively knew as a child. You will revel in knowing when to stop eating because you will return to feeling good after a meal.

To Eat Is Neat; but to Dine Is Divine

To eat is a necessity, but to eat intelligently is an art.
– Francois de la Rochefoucauld

When you eat, do it sitting at a table, doing nothing else. Eliminate distractions and don't read or watch TV. This allows you to enjoy the gift of fueling your body and helps you appreciate when you've had enough. When you're doing something else at the same time, you eat mindlessly, unaware of when you've had enough. One of my clients told me she had to eat with her eyes closed when she started doing this to keep her mind on eating.

Don't eat in the car. If you feel too busy to stop and eat, maybe you should slow down a pace or two. Or maybe you're really not hungry enough to take the time to stop and eat. And if you've trained yourself to associate driving with snacking, it's a habit worth breaking.

Take time to lovingly nurture your relationship with food. It is a lifelong relationship!

Incorporating Your Food Codes into Your Daily Routine

Keep a list of your best foods with you at all times. Stash a copy at work, in your gym locker, in your briefcase, and anywhere you might need it, so you can easily refer to it when you stop at the store or decide to eat out. But if you get separated from it you can always use muscle-testing on the fly.

If you don't like to cook or truly don't have time, you can buy prepared foods using your Food Codes plan or muscle-testing to find items that have the most value for you. Consider fresh and organic selections to reduce the toxic load on your body. A prepared rotisserie chicken from the grocery store is healthier than a bag of frozen chicken nuggets. Both are chicken, but the nuggets have been highly processed and contain many more additives.

Retest Seasonally and for Specific Needs

Your food requirements change according to your body's current needs and your reactions to stressors and conditions in your environment. As mentioned above, the changing of the seasons can stress your body. Other factors that influence the needs of your body include health conditions, age, gender, pregnancy, physical work load, the type of work you do, and the toxins you're exposed to. You might be exposed to toxins such as smoke, chemicals, and exhaust at your workplace.

For these reasons I suggest retesting your food lists every season – roughly every three months – even if you live where there is little change in conditions from season to season. This keeps you on a quarterly schedule. Or start with the new year and retest at the first of April, July, and October. Anything that helps you remember to retest about four times a year works.

And there's nothing wrong with retesting more often. If you have a bad cold or virus, ask your body what foods would be especially healing for you and for how many days you should consume them. If you are under extreme stress at your job, have a family issue, or even a tragedy in your community, test to see if you need any changes to your diet.

Other Ways to Use Muscle-Testing and the Food Codes

Keep in mind that the Food Codes method is not a diet as understood in the way most of us use the word. It is intended to help you know what foods will help balance your body's energy right now. The Food Codes is about using the energy of food to balance the energetic body you live in.

That said, there are various ways you can tailor your Food Codes to specific needs. You can find the best foods for a cleanse, to lose weight, for athletic training, for a health condition, or just for today – whatever "today" entails. You can test a particular combination of foods, and whether certain foods should *not* be eaten together. Keep in mind that dieting truths and systems you have followed in the past might not be true for you right now. Whatever your needs are, you now know how to determine what to eat for health and energy.

Paulina's Story

Paulina had problems with her bowel, chronic constipation, and bad sinus issues. She lived in a beautiful place and grew her own vegetables and herbs, had fruit bushes, and picked wild herbs in the meadows at the foot of the Alps. She was doing everything she could think of to improve her health.

She had stopped eating animal protein and was eating eggs for protein. When we tested for her best foods, eggs tested as one of her lowest-energy foods. Some of her highest-energy foods were Swiss cheese (which she had never heard of in her country), sardines, and salmon. She had loved sardines all her life yet had stopped eating them when she read articles that warned against eating fish. She had once hated broccoli yet came to really like it steamed with a sprinkle of Swiss cheese. Cottage cheese blended with flax seed oil; ground, fresh flax seeds; and fresh berries from her garden became a daily breakfast.

Wheat was not a good food for her, but wheat bran tested very high for several weeks. Simply mixing wheat bran with water and drinking it seemed to help ease her bowel problems, along with the flax seeds and cottage cheese mixture.

Paulina's doctor was really pleased by her progress in easing her constipation. Her protein deficiency resolved and she was encouraged to keep eating in this new way.

She noticed that she was becoming more intuitive as she learned to test her foods. She just started to know what foods were best for her. The foods that she needed started to "come to mind," and she would feel a strong desire to eat those foods.

She also learned an energy technique, "The 30-Second Gut Flush," for better digestion, which I will teach you in a later chapter. She did the Gut Flush several times daily, which eased the bloating in her abdomen. She noticed that her breathing was better, and her sinuses stopped dripping. In the spring she was able to get out and walk the beautiful hillsides with more "expanded breaths," as she put it.

Muscle-Testing for Your Family Members

You can use muscle-testing to determine the best foods for your loved ones. Ask the same questions you use to test yourself, substituting the other person's name for "I" and "me."

I did extensive testing when Bruce was in the hospital after his aneurysm and was able to supplement his diet to support his healing. You can even use this technique when your child has the flu. It really is a wonderful gift to give yourself and your family.

Your family members won't test best for the same foods, but you will have some best foods in common. Compare your family members' food lists. Use a blank Food Codes Food List and mark the foods you have in common. (See the "Cooking and Recipes" section for more about feeding your family.)

Don't Shop till You Drop

Shopping can be exhausting, and a couple of the top reasons for not eating well are not knowing what foods to buy and not having the time to read labels and shop selectively. Looking at every label on the shelf is impossible. And then there's the produce aisle, piled high with a quandary of fruits and vegetables.

Using your inner knower as a guide for shopping is fast, easy, discreet, and saves money. Use muscle-testing to test everything you put into your shopping cart. You can test any products you use in your home.

Kayla's Story

Kayla, a client in her early twenties, uses muscle-testing when she shops. She and her mom were grocery shopping together and tested their groceries as they went through the aisles. They hadn't noticed that they had caught the attention of another shopper. They were almost finished when a woman came up to them and said she had been watching them as they selected their groceries and she was very curious about what they were doing.

Right there in the grocery aisle, Kayla showed her how to muscle-test her groceries, and they tested the groceries in her cart. About half her groceries tested not good for her. She was flabbergasted and set off to put half her groceries back on the shelves.

Grocery-Testing Tips

Take your list of best foods and a combined list of your family's best foods with you as guides while grocery shopping, but muscle-test anything you're not sure about. Foods can test differently every time you shop. Sometimes organic foods test high and sometimes they don't. Some brands test higher than others for the same product. And some products of a particular brand test higher than others from the same brand.

In the produce aisle, test to see if variety matters. For example, test the different varieties of apples, and even individual apples. I always see people picking through the fruits and vegetables, squeezing and looking them over, so don't worry about anyone thinking you're too picky.

Do the same with packaged and canned foods. For foods such as canned tomatoes and beans, for which there are often many shelves of choices, zero in on what's best for you by testing one shelf or variety at a time, narrowing them down until you get to the best choice for you. For example, ask, "Are my best tomatoes on shelf two?" Then, "Of those on shelf two, are my best tomatoes whole or crushed? Then, "Is this brand of whole tomatoes best?" You can use these testing ideas at farmers' markets and anywhere else.

Several years ago, Bruce had a cold and was feeling under the weather. I thought he might need some specific foods, so I made a quick trip to the grocery store. I wanted to see how fast I could find the foods and nutrition he needed to help him feel better. From the entrance to the store I tested which section to go to first and went there. Then I tested which side of the aisle the food was on. Then I tested which section of the aisle the food was in. Then I tested which shelf the food was on. Then I quickly tested each food on that shelf to see which one it was.

I did this quickly through the store and came up with five foods Bruce needed to feel better. And they all made sense. I was at the checkout counter in six minutes! You can do this, too, with a little practice.

Eating Out

You can eat out very easily using muscle-testing. Before you leave you can test for the best place to eat. This is especially useful when you're traveling and don't know where to go. You have your trusty Food Codes plan with you at all times, so just refer to it when you order and/or muscle-test for the best foods on the menu. Most of the time there are several different meals that align with your plan.

Let's say that among your best foods are a variety of greens, vegetables, chicken, fish, butter, olive oil, and maybe sourdough bread. Think of all the options on a menu that you could eat based on just those foods. If the chef's salad comes close, but cheese and eggs are not at the top of your list right now, simply ask your server to omit the cheese and eggs. The house dressing with oil, vinegar, and spices also works. Most eating establishments are very willing to please and will customize your order on the spot.

When I find several dishes on a menu that test good for me I ask, "Will I enjoy the chef's salad the most?" or "Will the alfredo give me the most energy?" You can ask which meal will keep you on track with your weight loss.

One of my clients traveled five days a week for work and ate every meal out while he was away. He found a certain fast food restaurant that had a meal item made from his best foods. He was able to get a quick, easy meal that tested good for him there. It supported his weight loss of over fifty pounds.

You can test everything on a menu including water and drinks, and even with or without ice. Don't forget desserts, because a dessert might just test as divine!

CHAPTER 8

Improving the Way Your Body Uses Food

Now that you've learned how to access the wisdom of your inner knower to know exactly what to eat, there are some additional things you can do to support your glowing good health. Food is a key building block for a healthy body, yet we must consume other things like air, water, and sunshine for true radiant living.

First, Breathe

Eastern traditions include attention to the breath, and this focus is now being integrated into Western culture. Some years ago, we were visiting our son at college one weekend and took him to breakfast. After we finished breakfast we noticed a poster stuck up in the entryway of the cafe. It was just words on a pink sheet of paper advertising "Breathing Class." Our son was quite amused. "Really? Someone is teaching people how to breathe? Aren't we all doing that naturally?" he joked.

Actually, most of us take breathing for granted. We often breathe shallowly and don't give our bodies the oxygen they require. Just as food and water are nutrition for our bodies, so is air. Oxygen is a nutrient for humans, plants, and animals.

> *Spirit is a low flame inside us just waiting for the pump to bring the oxygen in. Outside circumstances do not activate the pump. We do. We can pump it any time we want.*
>
> *That's why taking a deep breath always improves any circumstance we are in. It dilutes fear and it focuses the mind. It relaxes the body and expands thinking, so it feeds the spirit. The word "inspire" literally means to "breathe in."*
>
> –Steve Chandler

Our lungs are an amazing duo. The respiratory system works to supply the entire body with oxygenated blood through breathing. With the help of the diaphragm we inhale oxygen and exhale carbon dioxide. The right lung has three lobes, while the left lung is a bit smaller, consisting of only two lobes, which allows a little more space in the chest for the heart. Together they contain about 1,500 miles of airways and 300 to 500 million alveoli, which are small, spongy, air-filled sacs attached to the branches of the bronchial tubes, the airways of the lungs. (https://en.wikipedia.org/wiki/Lung)

Improper breathing can distort our bodies physically as well as emotionally, mentally, and spiritually. Have you ever noticed that when you are stressed or worried you scarcely move any air? Most of us hold our breath in those moments, cutting off our supply of oxygen.

Muscle-Testing for Breathing and Oxygen Intake

Ask:

- On a scale of 0 to 10, how well am I breathing? 0? 1? 2? [etc.]
- On a scale of 0 to 10, how well am I taking in oxygen? 0? 1? 2? [etc.]

Your body is designed to detoxify about 70 percent of airborne toxins through breathing. Did that make you take a deep breath?

Relax and take another nice deep breath, pulling it way down to the bottom of your lungs and into your belly. Your shoulders should not move up – keep them relaxed – and breathe out. Now take three normal breaths. Hopefully you're feeling more centered and calm.

Muscle-Testing for Improved Breathing

Retest your breathing for improvement by asking:

- How well am I breathing now on a scale of 0 to 10? 0? 1? 2? [etc.]
- How well am I taking in oxygen now on a scale of 0 to 10? 0? 1? 2? [etc.]

You might find quite a difference from before you concentrated on your breathing.

There are many kinds of breathing exercises, and you can test to see if there is a particular method that is best for you. Or you can simply give yourself an instant energy boost of nutritious oxygen by breathing deeply! Try taking several deep breaths at the top of each hour. It's easy and provides instant relaxation as well as more energy and clearer thinking. Post a reminder where you will see it often or set a timer on your phone.

Conscious breathing can help relieve pain, increase lymph and blood circulation, strengthen organs and core muscles, help you sleep better, and so much more. While you're learning the muscle-testing techniques and still feeling a little uncertain about them, take several nice deep breaths before you begin testing. It really helps!

The Nutrient of Water

> *As our bodies are mostly made of water, I'd rather be hungry than thirsty. And as love is mostly made up of sugar water, I'd rather be a hummingbird caged in your heart.*
> *– Jarod Kintz*

We are not just what we eat; we are also what we drink. Humans can survive for several weeks without food, but water is a different story; we can't survive long without it. With no water in hot conditions we become out of balance and fall into dehydration in about an hour. Within seventy-two hours, even in good conditions, we go into shock and fall into a comatose state. (http://www.businessinsider.com/how-many-days-can-you-survive-without-water-2014-5)

Dehydration is when more water is leaving the body than is coming in. We lose water through breathing, sweat, urine, and feces. In hot conditions an adult can sweat about 1.5 liters of water in a few hours. (M. L. Sawka et al, "Thermoregulatory responses to acute exercise-heat stress and heat acclimation," in M. J. Fregly & C. M. Blatteis's *Handbook of Physiology. Section 4: Environmental Physiology*, (New York: Oxford University Press, 1996), ISBN 0-19-507492-0) People even sweat when they're in the water. Maybe you remember becoming thirsty while swimming, even though you were in the water.

When people call me to get help with headaches, pain, dizziness, and flu-like symptoms, I often find that the only problem is dehydration – easily cured by drinking a few glasses of water. Mild dehydration can cause dizziness, headache, drowsiness, blurry sight, weakness, heart palpitations, muscle cramps, and many more symptoms. Chronic dehydration can lead to pain and eventually degenerative disease.

Water is a life-giving miracle. Water crosses our cell membranes freely, but we need to maintain good hydration to take care of our wonderful body parts.

Fruits and vegetables are loaded with water. A cucumber is almost 90 percent water – a fantastic source of water and a delicious hydrating snack. You can carry a cucumber with you like a water bottle with edible packaging. Watermelon, berries, tomatoes, peppers, and apples are full of natural, nutrient-packed water. Lettuce and greens are mostly water. Think of the weight of fruits and vegetables. That weight is from their water content.

Judith's Story

Judith was a legal assistant at a busy law firm on the East Coast. She was in her mid-fifties and had received diagnoses of fibromyalgia and chronic fatigue syndrome. She took a leave of absence and came to our clinic because she could barely work anymore. She was in such pain that she had trouble walking. She had moved in with her elderly mother so her mother could help take care of her!

We found that Judith had severe dehydration. She was very overweight, but most of it was water. She was holding about forty pounds of excess water weight in her body, her body's attempt to keep electrolytes and other nutrients dissolved. Her body was trying to keep dangerous toxins from becoming concentrated and causing symptoms of toxicity. Toxins were coming from parasites, the toxic waste they excrete, and heavy metals.

When I asked how much water she drank daily, she replied, "None." She went on to say that she drank a gallon of coffee every day to keep herself going. An entire gallon! She ate a lot of donuts at the office, fast food, and an occasional salad, but no water.

Muscle-testing revealed that the most important foods for Judith were greens, cabbage, leafy lettuce, fresh tomatoes, apples, watermelon, pineapple, and tuna. She also needed to drink steam-distilled water to help clear toxins from her body.

It wasn't surprising to us that coffee did not test high for her. She actually had an intolerant reaction to coffee that made her very tired rather than providing the energy she was trying to get from it.

Judith's mother made fresh vegetable soups and stir-fried and sautéed cabbage and greens. Tuna salad with chopped celery and apples over fresh lettuce and spinach became one of her favorite salad staples. Tomato juice and vegetable juice replaced the coffee, along with steam-distilled water.

Judith was amazed by how quickly her energy returned once she started eating the foods her body really needed to heal. She shed weight and felt like a new woman. While Judith was recovering, she decided to extend her leave of absence and enjoy life with her renewed energy. She took a vacation in Mexico with her daughter and later was able to return to her career.

Water is needed to filter your blood, support kidney and liver function, and produce urine. When you don't drink enough water, your body retains fat and water around your midsection. Drinking sufficient water and eating water-rich foods balances your body's store of water; hydrates your skin, improving skin tone and appearance; and hydrates your muscles, helping them function optimally and clear out toxins after exercising.

Between earth and earth's atmosphere, the amount of water remains constant; there is never a drop more, never a drop less. This is a story of circular infinity.
– Linda Hogan

But all water is not created equal. Maybe it was in the beginning, but no longer. It is no secret that water pollution is a worldwide problem. Pollutants have been found in waters thought to be untouched and pristine in the far reaches of the planet. Newspaper articles have circulated about the 60,000 different chemicals used in farming and industry that can get into our water supply. Water is treated with chemicals added for "safety," such as fluoride to harden teeth.

Water filters are very popular today for this very reason. My family lives in an area that claims to have some of the purest water in the world. It comes from a deep well and tastes great. One day a patient came to the office for a treatment. He had been fixing a broken water pipe not far from our home. I commented on how great our water is and how lucky we are to not be on a big city water system. He scoffed and said, "Are you kidding? You should see the slime in those pipes! I won't drink it!" We got a water filtration system right away!

Just how good for you is that expensive bottled water that comes from a "pure spring" thousands of miles away? Your tap water is likely subject to more stringent testing and quality regulation. Use-and-toss bottled water is not the answer. We don't need any more plastic bottles in our landfills or ending up in our waterways. The UN reports that more than 8 million tons of garbage is dumped into the ocean every year. (http://web.unep.org/unepmap/un-declares-war-ocean-plastic) Many plastic products, from sippy cups to food wraps, release chemicals that act like the hormone estrogen when ingested. Tap water is cleaner, less expensive, and thus healthier, according to the National Resource Defense Counsel. (https://www.nrdc.org/stories/truth-about-tap)

That is not to say that all tap water meets regulatory standards, however. If you have concerns about the quality of your tap water, simply use a water filtration system. There are many types of water filters available in a wide range of prices, from filtering pitchers to large systems that filter all the water in your house. You can use muscle-testing to determine whether your tap water is healthy for you or you should use a filtration system.

Do I Need to Drink Eight Glasses a Day?

You've probably heard of the "8x8 rule" – that you should drink eight 8-ounce glasses of water each day for good health. According to Mayo Clinic, "For your body to function properly, you must replenish its water supply by consuming beverages and foods that contain water." (https://www.mayoclinic.org/healthy-lifestyle/nutrition-and-healthy-eating/in-depth/water/art-20044256) And the Institute of Medicine determined that an adequate intake for men is roughly three liters (about 13 cups) of total beverages a day, and for women it's 2.2 liters (about 9 cups). (http://www8.nationalacademies.org/onpinews/newsitem.aspx?RecordID=10925)

Although the 8x8 rule doesn't exactly match the Institute of Medicine's recommendation, it remains popular because it's easy to remember.

Yet there is disagreement in the scientific community about how much water we should consume. You've probably read articles that contradicted each other. Barbara Rolls, Professor of Nutrition Sciences at Pennsylvania State University, said, "Water requirements depend so much on outside temperature, activity levels and other factors that there isn't one rule that fits everybody." (Dan Negoianu and Stanley Goldfarb, "Just Add Water," *Journal of the American Society of Nephrology*, 2008, http://jasn.asnjournals.org/content/19/6/1041.full) Research done by Professor Stanley Goldfarb, physician and nephrologist at the University of Pennsylvania, and colleagues, as reported in the same article cited above, found:

There is no clear evidence of benefit from drinking increased amounts of water. Although we wish we could demolish all of the urban myths found on the Internet regarding the benefits of supplemental water ingestion, we concede there is also no clear evidence of *lack* of benefit. In fact, there is simply a lack of evidence in general.

It is known that drinking alcohol dehydrates the body, and too much coffee or black tea has a diuretic effect on the kidneys, though there is disagreement about whether this is detrimental to health. So it's important to include plain water in your fluid intake. And foods with high water content may hydrate your body better at times than water. Water-rich fruits and vegetables like watermelon, celery, and cucumber are like food and drink combined. They provide minerals, natural salts, sugars, vitamins, amino acids, and nutrients that have yet to be discovered. Soups, stews, and broths are loaded with a bounty of nutrition and hydrating nutrients. Our mothers and grandmothers knew this and used carcasses and leftovers to make nutritious broths and soups. Sipping a mug of vegetable or bone broth has beneficial hydrating qualities as well as being nutritious and delicious.

The perplexing question is, how can you know how much water and liquid you need and what kind of water is best for you? By now you know the answer:

Muscle-Testing for Hydration

Ask:
- Am I taking in enough liquids?
- Are there certain hydrating foods that I need at this time? (Look to your Food Codes for guidance.)
- Am I drinking enough water?
- How much water do I need to drink daily? Six cups? Eight cups? Ten cups? [etc.] (This varies more often than food requirements, so ask often.)
- Am I drinking the right kind of water? (If the answer is no, ask what kind of water is best.)

Improving the Way Your Body Uses Food

- Is the water in my home okay to drink? (If no, look into filtering your water, and muscle-test for what kind of filter to purchase.)
- Is it okay for me to drink with meals?
- Is water with ice okay?

Ask any other questions you have about water. If you drink water from sources other than your home, such as water delivered from a water company, muscle-test that water as well.

Dehydration can have several underlying causes even if you are taking in the right kinds and the right amounts of liquids. Toxins and pathogens can cause dehydration, and they can be an underlying cause of water retention as well.

Water is called the universal solvent because it can dissolve substances better than any other liquid. Consider the Grand Canyon carved deep into the crust of the earth by flowing water. Water is important as a solvent in your body because it transports valuable nutrients, chemicals, and minerals throughout your body as well as transporting toxic substances out of your body. It is imperative for good circulation, a powerful healer, and the most important nutrient for every living thing on the planet.

> *Nothing is softer or more flexible than water,*
> *yet nothing can resist it.*
> *– Lao Tzu*

Diane's Story

Using the Food Codes plan I have noticed that my stomach doesn't have so many issues since I have eliminated my "no" foods. I used to have diarrhea quite frequently and lots of bloating. I also have lost eight pounds in the past few weeks and my sleep is much deeper. Overall, I feel more energy in the afternoon and I don't fall into the 3pm zombie mode anymore.

I used to love my wine. On my Food Codes plan alcohol is a "no" for me, so wine is not one of my good foods. I stopped drinking it. Recently I have discovered that I have zero tolerance to alcohol and I have lost the desire for alcohol altogether. I have an expensive bottle of wine that I have been saving for a special occasion and I am going to just give it away.

I highly recommend that people have their food sensitivity evaluated using the Food Codes method to up-level their health and vitality!

Supplements

Nutritional guidelines are very broad and formulated for the general population, not for each individual person. As with food, only your body knows how much of certain nutrients you need. You are a unique individual whose nutritional needs vary from those others. No hodgepodge of isolated vitamins thrown together in a box of "functional food" is ideal for anyone's specific nutritional needs.

Western culture has trained us to take medicine and drugs. With this training we take vitamins in the same way we take drugs, assuming they will improve how we feel. We think that vitamins are totally safe, and if a little is good, well... more just might be better. This is not true.

As is the case with all dietary supplements, the decision to use supplemental vitamins should not be taken lightly, according to Dr. Vasilios Frankos, the director of the Federal Drug Administration's Division of Dietary Supplement Programs. He said, "Vitamins are not dangerous unless you get too much of them," and "More is not necessarily better with supplements, especially if you take fat-soluble vitamins." (https://www.fda.gov/ForConsumers/ConsumerUpdates/ucm118079.htm)

Most people don't ingest megadoses of supplements, but if you eat a fortified cereal at breakfast, grab an energy bar between meals, have enriched pasta for dinner, and take a daily supplement, you could easily be over the recommended daily intake of a host of nutrients. Chances are the unfortified foods you eat aren't a problem. "It's pretty hard to overdo it from food alone," said Johanna Dwyer, RD, a senior research scientist with the National Institutes of Health's Office of Dietary Supplements. "Most people don't realize there's no real advantage to taking more than the recommended amounts of vitamins and minerals, and they don't recognize there may be disadvantages," Dwyer said. For example, too much selenium can lead to hair loss, bowel upset, fatigue, and nerve damage. Too much vitamin C or zinc can cause diarrhea, stomach upset, and nausea. (https://www.quora.com/Can-you-eat-too-many-health-foods-or-take-too-many-supplements)

Mandi's Story

The nutritional Food Codes plan has made a significant difference in my life. It has allowed me to truly enjoy the foods I eat because I know they are what my body needs, and I know that my body is getting the nutrients it needs from these foods.

I have since been able to stop my multivitamin, I am feeling happier, less anxious, and I am sleeping better through the night.

Thank you, Lana, for helping me to feel well and be well with the food plan and your energetic gifts!

Lara's Story

Lara came to the clinic pale and exhausted. She had heavy periods with excessive bleeding. We found that she had a major problem with parasites, which rob the body of nutrients and minerals like iron.

Lara was very deficient in iron, but had an overabundance of iron as well. Excess iron is usually stored in the liver, heart, and pancreas. Lara had heart palpitations and worried that she had a heart problem. The problem was that her body could not absorb new sources of iron until it got rid of the old iron being held in the cells of her organs, so she actually had an iron deficiency.

She took a homeopathic remedy that helped release the excess iron from her organs' cells. She also did the 30-Second Gut Flush daily to help clear out excess toxins. (You will learn the gut flush in the following chapter.)

Her food plan revealed that red meat, greens, and beets were some of her top foods. Her local butcher stocked fresh organic liver, and she found that she loved lightly fried liver and onions. She also needed to take a natural, food-based iron supplement for a short time to replenish her body, and herbal supplements to help expel the parasites.

Lara did well with this plan and has had no more problems with iron deficiency or excess. She said that she can now walk up the stairs without having to stop and rest in the middle.

Minerals are another source of controversy among health care professionals. Over seventy minerals are needed by the body. There are two kinds of minerals, organic and inorganic, and they are structurally different. Plants break down inorganic minerals in the soil for their use and change them into organic minerals. Organic minerals are obtained from plants and are more easily absorbed by the body's cells than inorganic ones. This is one of the reasons why good fruits and vegetables are so beneficial for our bodies.

There are nutrients called "essential" and "non-essential." You've probably heard the terms *essential vitamins*, *essential amino acids*, and *essential minerals*. These are nutrients that the body needs to function that cannot be made in the body and must be obtained from food. Only your unique body knows what is "essential" for you. Eating whole foods instead of processed foods helps provide your body with the nutrients it needs. It was designed to utilize the whole, complete nutrition contained in whole foods.

The nutrients discovered to date might not be even a thimbleful of all the nutrients our bodies use. We need a nice variety of real, whole foods that test high on our individual Food Codes lists. Our bodies are wise and know what to do with the multitude of nutrients available in plants and animals. They use the best and excrete the rest.

> *As for butter versus margarine,*
> *I trust cows more than chemists.*
> – Joan Gussow

With news of depleted soils and questions about the nutritional quality of foods, do you need nutritional supplements? Some professionals say you should have your blood tested periodically to see if you're maintaining the proper levels of certain vitamins and nutrients, and some say it's not necessary. You now know that your body knows the answers to these questions.

Muscle-Testing for the Need for Supplements

Ask: "Do I need to supplement my diet with nutritional supplements at this time?"

Sunshine

Without sunshine this planet would be lifeless. Some cultures worship the sun, some fear it, and some think it causes disease. Some scientists have labeled it harmful because it causes cancer, while others report that a million people die every year from lack of exposure to sunshine.

Sunshine gives life to plants and animals and I consider it a nutrient for the body and soul. Its benefits reach far beyond the production of vitamin D. It can help heal many conditions including wounds, skin conditions, and infections, and actually protects *against* melanoma.

Sunshine can sterilize and disinfect, killing disease-causing germs. It is beneficial for depression and brain function, skin and bone health, asthma, blood pressure, and blood oxygen content, and enhances the immune system. It helps lower cholesterol and purifies and detoxifies the body. It can help you sleep better and can even help children grow taller.

Too much of a good thing, be it food, exercise, or sunshine, is just that – too much. Be wise about your exposure to sunshine and you will reap many benefits from it. Just as you wouldn't attempt a marathon if you hadn't trained for it gradually, exposing yourself to the sun gradually is key.

Muscle-Testing for Sun Exposure

Ask:

- Do I need more sunshine?
- Should I use sunscreen?
- Is [brand, type, or SPF factor] sunscreen good for me?

Exercise

Ask ten experts what kind of exercise is best, and you will get ten different answers. Have you been told that you must get moving and exercise to lose weight? Have you been told that exercising will boost your metabolism and give you more energy? Both these recommendations can be true or totally false. You are led to believe that you need to force your body to exercise when the truth is that you might actually need more rest. Forcing your body to exercise when it needs to rest can cause exhaustion and energy depletion. You already know that your body knows best.

A few years ago, I read in a magazine that climbing stairs is the best way to get in shape. I lived in a three-story home so I had two flights of stairs just waiting to get me in shape! I didn't need to join a gym! So I started right away. I bounded up and down those stairs and it felt great! I slowed down when I started to get tired, but I kept pushing myself to keep going. "Shape up, Girl!" I said to myself.

I could barely walk for the next several days.

So the message is to start gently and easily with any kind of exercise. You can map out an exercise plan using muscle-testing, but keep in mind your other daily needs and your ever-changing environmental stresses. After a tough day at work you could need either a nice jog or a fifteen-minute nap on the couch.

Take it from me: don't try to get yourself in shape in one day. If you need more physical exercise, start slowly and gradually.

Muscle-Testing for the Need for Exercise

Ask:

- Do I need to exercise?
- Do I need more exercise than I currently get?
- Do I need different exercise than what I am doing currently?
- Do I need [general, endurance, strength, etc. (see chart below)]?
- Do I need [walking, aerobic dance, circuit training, etc. (see chart below for exercises in the category determined above)]?
- Should I [walk, dance, weight-train, etc.] [once a week? twice a week? three times a week? etc.]

Improving the Way Your Body Uses Food

Exercise Chart

General exercise	Walking
	Hiking
	Mini-trampoline/Rebounding
	Pilates
	Treadmill
	Water exercise or water aerobics
	Other
Endurance (to increase heart rate and breathing)	Aerobics
	Aerobic dance
	Basketball
	Biking
	Stationary cycling
	Brisk walking
	Dancing/Zumba
	Jogging
	Jump-roping
	Running
	Swimming laps
	Stair-climbing/Hill-climbing
	Tennis
	Yard work (push-mowing, raking, digging)
	Other
Strength (to make muscles stronger)	Circuit training (high-intensity exercise)
	Using a resistance band to build muscles
	Weight-lifting
	Push-ups
	Planks
	Other

Balance (to improve balance, strength, and brain fitness)	Tai chi Standing on one foot Heal-to-toe walking Ballet Balance board/Wobble board Exercise ball Other
Flexibility (to stretch muscles, stay limber, improve mobility)	Stretching Yoga Restorative yoga Other
Rest	Stay quiet and still Concentrate on breathing Morning nap (how long?) Afternoon nap (how long?) Other
Meditation (to reduce stress, anxiety, pain, or fatigue, or nurture your soul)	Transcendental meditation Zen meditation Walking meditation Mindfulness meditation Self-inquiry Prayer

The bottom line is that you don't have to wonder and worry about how much water to drink or what supplements to take or what kind of exercise is best. Take a deep breath and relax, knowing that you can just ask your inner knower and use your favorite muscle-testing method to find the answer. You'll find a list of common vitamins and minerals in the Food Codes Food List. Test them just as you test for foods, and your body will tell you exactly what is needed.

CHAPTER 9
Feeling Great All the Time

Now, good digestion wait on appetite, And health on both!
– William Shakespeare

Hunger

Many of us eat for comfort. When we are upset, angry, bored, or frightened, we eat to feel better. Food numbs us and gives us a momentary bit of pleasure – until we notice we've eaten a tub of ice cream or a full sleeve of Thin Mints. Then we feel guilty on top of the original uncomfortable feeling that started the process.

Emotions impact eating and controlling weight for many, especially women. Perhaps it is because we were raised to be pleasant and kind, so we stuff our emotions deep inside and keep them there with our food.

Eating addictions, bingeing, and non-stop eating have causes from intense emotions to neurological imbalances. You find yourself constantly hungry even when you're full, and you just can't stop eating. You head to the store at night in your jammies to get chips and ice cream and rip into the bag of chips as you drive home.

If you're standing in front of the refrigerator feeling desperate to eat something when you don't think you should be hungry, pause, take a deep breath, and use your muscle-testing:

Muscle-Testing for Hunger and Thirst

Ask:

- On a scale of 0 to 10, how hungry am I right now? 0? 1? 2? [etc.]
- On a scale of 0 to 10, how thirsty am I right now? 0? 1? 2? [etc.]

If you rate yourself high for hunger or thirst, first drink a big glass of water and relax for a moment. The need for water can make you feel hungry and satisfying that need quells the hungry feeling. If you still feel hungry, have something on your food plan and enjoy it fully! If you didn't test high for hunger or thirst, you might be emotionally hungry.

Blocks to Healthy Eating

Writer's block is when you are totally stuck and cannot write a sentence. Similar blocks can keep you from doing lots of things, and emotions are often the cause. They can even be at the root of physical blocks to health and they can block healthy eating, keeping you stuck in unhealthy eating patterns ranging from overeating to starving yourself.

A block can deflect your energy toward a negative path, such as grabbing a candy bar instead of a good food on your food plan. A block can make you rationalize negative thinking like "Healthy foods cost too much," "I don't like health food," and "I don't have time to eat healthy." How about this block?: "I'll never be able to change how I eat." To have a better relationship with healthy eating and get rid of such negative thinking, do the easy meditation and clearing exercise below. It takes about ten minutes and can bring you profound understanding of your blocks and help you clear any you discover.

Energy-Balancing Exercise for Hunger and Thirst

Have paper and pen handy, and a magnet if you have one. During the exercise write down the impressions that come to mind.

Step 1: Discover the block.

a. Sit comfortably and relax.

b. Take a few deep breaths and relax even more as you notice your breathing. Let your shoulders drop and your tummy soften. Close your eyes if that helps you relax more.

c. Ask, "Do I have a block associated with healthy eating?" If yes, write down as many things as you can think of.

d. Choose the block that feels the strongest and move to step 2. If no block revealed itself, move to step 2 using "I have a block to healthy eating" as your block.

Step 2: Clear the block.

a. Muscle-test for how strong the block feels on a scale of 0 to 10, and write down the number.

b. Use a magnet, the palm of your hand, or your fingertips to swipe the top of your head from front to back while saying or thinking, "I release [name of block]. (If you are doing this for another person, swipe down their back.) Do this three or more times.

c. Take a nice deep breath.

d. Again, muscle-test for how strong the block feels on a scale of 0 to 10, and write down the number.

e. If the block has cleared, you can do this again with another block. If the block still rates high, continue clearing and rechecking until you feel like the block has diminished or released.

Most people notice that they feel neutral about the block after doing this exercise, and that naming their block now feels silly or even ridiculous. You can do this exercise over and over with other thoughts or problems you have regarding your relationship to healthy eating.

If emotional or uncontrollable eating is a problem you can't clear on your own, go to TheFoodCodes.com for additional information on combining The Food Codes with The Emotion Code.

Digest Your Food Properly

Food is all those substances which, submitted to the action of the stomach, can be assimilated or changed into life by digestion, and can thus repair the losses which the human body suffers through the act of living.
– Jean Anthelme Brillat-Savarin

Our bodies are marvelous creations. They really are temples. So many things happen in them without any effort on our part. Just imagine if you had to tell your lungs to breathe, your blood to circulate, or your stomach to empty.

The process of digestion is complex, miraculous, and awesome, and involves many internal organs, yet it normally functions without any supervision. The gut has been called our second brain. Every morsel, spoonful, tiny taste, drink, gulp, quick swallow, or breath of air has to be digested, assimilated, or eliminated. The gut is eventually involved in doing the same for everything we rub, smear, spritz, sniff, drop, apply, or inject on or into our skin, hair, eyes, ears, nose, and nails.

Good digestion is essential to our well-being. Our bodies are marvels that we take for granted most of the time as they keep on functioning on automatic pilot, year after year. But many of us experience digestive problems and chronic digestive pain that make us sit up and pay attention. Pain is the signal that something is not right. Medicating pain that is trying to alert us to a problem, is like killing the messenger.

> *It has long been known for sure that the sight of tasty food makes a hungry man's mouth water.*
> *– Ivan Pavlov*

Digestion begins even before you open your mouth to pop in a morsel. It starts with a simple thought about food in your brain, whether sneaking a bite or planning a whole meal. The aroma and sight of the food further ignite your digestive engine. You eat with your head your eyes, and your nose, before you eat with your mouth.

How Digestion Works

Brain: Your brain flashes electrical alerts to turn on the digestive system. Have you ever uttered, "Yummm," while surfing through the delectable pictures in a food magazine?

Mouth: One of the first physical changes is your mouth salivating and your enzymes starting to flow. Just thinking about biting into a fresh, juicy lemon makes your salivary glands burst with a flood of saliva. A bite of food is put into your mouth and ground up by the teeth, and saliva starts to break it down from a solid to a liquid.

Esophagus: Chewed food (hopefully well-chewed food) is swallowed with the help of your tongue pushing it back into your throat and down your esophagus. Automatic downward contractions in your esophagus steadily push the mixture toward your stomach.

Stomach: The cardiac sphincter valve at the beginning of your stomach — a ring-shaped muscle — opens and admits the food into your stomach. Then it closes to prevent food and acidic juices from being pushed back into your esophagus. Powerful digestive juices and acids mix with the food in your stomach before the mushy mixture exits through your pyloric sphincter valve, another ring-shaped muscle. This valve allows only a particular amount of food into your small intestine so that it won't overfill. It also keeps the food that has moved into your small intestine from returning to your stomach.

Liver: Your liver is your largest internal organ — about the size of a football, and weighs in at about three-and-a-half pounds. It is also your largest gland. It is a masterpiece of functions that help detoxify your body. You ingest a multitude of toxins daily that you are totally unaware of. Your liver is like a warehouse that stores glycogen — a form of sugar that converts to glucose, another form of sugar — to be used by your body when it needs it, including your muscles, brain, and central nervous system.

It produces bile, an alkaline compound that aids digestion and helps emulsify fats and lipids. It also secretes enzymes into the small intestine that assist with digestion and absorption of nutrients.

Gallbladder: Your gallbladder is a little organ about three inches long that sits under the right lobe of your liver. Bile, also known as gall, is stored here and released into the duodenum area of the upper small intestine to break down fats for absorption. After fat is absorbed, the bile returns to your liver to be reused.

Pancreas: Your pancreas is involved in blood sugar control and metabolism and secretes enzymes into your small intestine that assist with digestion and absorption of nutrients.

Small intestine: Stretched out like a hose, your small intestine would be fifteen to twenty feet long depending on how tall you are. It has three main sections: the duodenum, the jejunum, and the ileum, and is lined with finger-like projections called villi and microvilli. The surface area of your small intestine is roughly the size of a tennis court. Most food absorption takes place in the small intestine.

Ileocecal valve: Your ileocecal valve is located at the end of your small intestine. It opens and closes appropriately to allow digested food matter into your large intestine and keeps the contents of the large intestine from backing up. Each section of the digestive system has valves to stop the backflow of food and assist with the onward process of digestion.

Appendix: Your appendix is located at the junction of the small and large intestines. It is a "safe house" for good bacteria. In case of illness these good bacteria repopulate your gut.

Large intestine: By the time food gets to your large intestine, or colon, most of it has been absorbed by your body; hence the saying "You are what you eat." The liquid and remaining nutrients are absorbed through your colon tube, which is about five feet long and goes from your ileocecal valve at the lower right side of your torso upward to just under your ribs and continues across the top of your abdomen and turns downward in a sort of S curve to your rectum and anus.

Valves of Houston: John Houston, an Irish-British anatomist after whom these valves are named, was the first to describe them. They are three or four muscle flaps or folds on either side of your rectal wall, like steps, just above your anal canal. The folds support the weight of fecal matter and prevent it from surging toward the anus.

Anus: Continuing the digestive journey to the finish line of the anal canal, the anus muscle controls the expulsion of stool from your body.

It Takes Guts to Be Healthy

Billions of bacteria flourish in the large intestine – or should – for tip-top health and the best digestion. Undigested matter and a very large number of bacteria make up the stool or feces. Normal feces are composed of about 75 percent water and 25 percent solid matter. About 30 percent of that solid matter is dead bacteria.

The human body maintains a complex ecosystem of bacteria from the outside to the inside, mostly located in the gut, where it is called the microbiome. The study of the human microbiome is fascinating and is one of the fastest growing fields in medical research.

Not all bacteria are bad. The bacteria that colonize the surfaces and insides of our bodies are essential for life. We are completely dependent on "good" bacteria to help digest our food, produce certain vitamins, regulate strong immune systems, and keep us healthy. Our microbiomes appear to function almost like endocrine organs, helping other parts of our endocrine systems. Healthy gut bacteria equates to healthy bodies with fewer ailments.

As you can see, the digestive system is much more than a twenty-five-foot tube for funneling tasty substances through your body. Think about your miraculous digestive process the next time you enjoy food. Your body will be converting that food into your flesh and blood.

Almost 80 percent of your immune system is housed in your gut. Your enteric nervous system governs your digestive tract from your throat to your anus. This has been dubbed "the second brain," and it might be involved in "digesting" and processing emotional messages as well. You don't want your second brain to malfunction because it's clogged up!

Backed-Up Gut

Do you have belly fat, pain, heartburn, exhaustion, headaches, acid reflux, bad breath, constipation, sour stomach, gas, or diarrhea? If you do, you might have a backed-up gut. Toxins from unexpelled fecal matter can back up into your belly and the tissue of your arms, legs, and your whole body, even your brain. Add to these your own naturally produced metabolic waste, and environmental toxins from food, air, water, and products you use on your body, and the backup can become quite poisonous. It can leak into your bloodstream, organs, and glands. Skin rashes and sores are often signs of toxins and poisons coming out onto the skin. It is difficult to have bowel movements when fecal matter hardens and the waste gets backed up.

Digestive diseases are rampant in our society, such as gastroesophageal reflux disease, diverticulitis, inflammatory bowel disease, celiac disease, irritable bowel syndrome, Crohn's disease, ulcerative colitis, hemorrhoids, and many forms of cancer. These are the top six ways to avoid digestive diseases:

- Chew food thoroughly.
- Don't overeat. Ask your inner knower to tell you when to stop eating.
- Get plenty of fluids. Muscle-test to find out what your best fluids are and what amount of fluids is optimal for you.
- Eat foods that contain fiber. Muscle-test to find out if you need to eat more fiber-rich foods.
- Avoid aspirin, alcohol, and coffee, and don't smoke. Avoid foods, especially fats, that test below a 5 on your Food Codes plan.
- Exercise daily. Muscle-test to see what's the best exercise for you and how often you should exercise; and maybe you actually need more rest.

Andy's Story

Andy was a professional dancer and dance instructor in his late thirties. He started to lose strength in his legs and other muscles and was tired all the time. At first he didn't worry about it because he was working so hard; he thought it was normal to be so exhausted.

Then he started having brain fog, memory problems, panic attacks, and bouts of depression out of the blue. He was told that the panic attacks were all in his head and he simply needed to relax more. The muscle problems became worse to the point that it was hard to stand up straight. So he followed the advice and went to a beautiful tropical island, even though he wasn't able to hike and explore as he wanted to. He felt like an old man walking all hunched over and in pain.

His continued depression and increasing paranoia, caused him to become reclusive, and his muscle problems forced him to give up dancing.

Andy eventually found out through a doctor who was a heavy metals specialist, that he was very toxic. Concentrated amounts of aluminum, cadmium, and lead were backed up in his body. This made sense because he had been exposed to cigarette smoke since he had been a baby, as his parents were heavy smokers. Cigarette smoke contains cadmium, among other toxins. He rarely drank water. He drank mostly soda and beer from aluminum cans. His physician put him on a stringent detoxification program.

I worked with Andy to address his struggles with depression and panic attacks. We found that the heavy-metal toxins were his underlying problem, triggering what he thought were emotional issues. His body was not releasing toxins naturally as it should, due to his very poor digestive system.

We muscle-tested Andy's Food Codes and found his best foods. These included apples, pineapple, raisins, many green foods, cilantro, parsley, cooked cabbage, radishes, sea kelp, lemons, and vinegar. There were several "good for Andy" fats like olive oil, butter, beef fat, lard, and walnut oil.

Andy was retested for toxic levels by his physician after using his Food Codes plan for four months. His physician was surprised at the fast drop in levels of heavy metals, because detoxifying from heavy metal poisons can take years. He asked Andy what in the world he was doing; he hadn't seen this fast of a decline with anyone before. Andy told him that he was taking the detox protocol the physician had put him on and working with me using his Food Codes plan. The physician told him to definitely keep doing that. At Andy's most recent checkup, which found he was still improving, his physician asked for more details about the Food Codes.

Andy's life has turned around. The panic attacks are gone and his depression has lifted. He and his fiancée are planning a honeymoon to that beautiful tropical island he visited. They plan to explore it all on foot.

Health issues from heavy metals and industrial toxins are considered one of the top health concerns these days. Keeping your body's detoxification pathways open is a major must for your body, mind, and emotional health.

The 30-Second Gut Flush

This is an energy technique to keep your body and belly happy. This simple daily exercise encourages your body to remove fecal matter along with the toxins you ingest on a daily basis.

Ten benefits of the 30-Second Gut Flush:

1. Slim the belly and reduce belly fat
2. Increase oxygen in your body
3. Release bloating and gas
4. Better blood circulation
5. Stimulate organs, glands, lymph system, and chakras
6. Relax muscle tension around the bowel
7. Help dislodge or break up fecal matter
8. Improve brain communication
9. Help balance bodily systems
10. More effective than antacids and laxatives!

The Food Codes: Intuitive Eating for Every Body

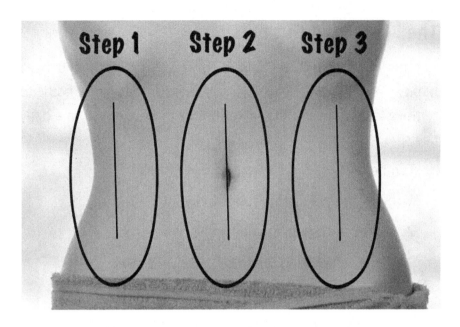

This exercise is easy to do lying down but can also be done standing or sitting.

1. Focus on your abdominal area from the bottom of your ribcage to the top of your groin and pelvic bone. Mentally divide this area into three parts:
    a. Under your right rib/breast to the top of your right hip bone
    b. Under the center of your sternum/breast bone to your pelvic/pubic bone
    c. Under your left rib/breast to the top of your left hip bone
2. Put the palm of your hand flat on the right-hand section with your fingers extended.
3. Take nice deep breaths as you rub the section with a light, downward sweep, performing ten sweeps on each section, moving right to left.

4. Keep breathing deeply as you do three sets of ten sweeps. Deep breathing helps clear toxins while oxygenating your brain and body.

You can watch a video of the Gut Flush technique at TheFoodCodes.com

Do the Gut Flush every morning before you get out of bed to start your day, and as you lie down at bedtime to balance yourself at the end of your day. You can also do it before and/or after meals to aid digestion. It is one of the easiest and most beneficial exercises of your day. You can do it when traveling and when sitting for long periods of time. A client told me she was waiting in the airport between flights and started feeling full and sluggish. She did the Gut Flush right there in the crowded airport and felt better quickly.

You can also use this technique on children and babies. Always use gentle, light strokes. You can stroke lightly with your fingertips. *Do not use pressure, jab, or poke!*

Children can do the Gut Flush by themselves. It's fun, and they often have tummy aches that can be relieved with this simple technique. Animals love this technique too. Help your pet's digestion and health with the Gut Flush, especially if they like having their belly rubbed.

The Gut Flush can also be performed without touching your body. Simply sweep your hand in the method shown without touching your body. The energy from your hand is very effective, especially when you have a skin rash or pain.

CHAPTER 10

Intentional Eating – The Art of Enjoying Your Food and Your Life

*Eating is really one of your indoor sports.
You play three times a day, and it's well worthwhile to
make the game as pleasant as possible.*
– Dorothy Draper

In this chapter I provide some tips to help you enjoy your food more fully. Now that you know how to use the Food Codes muscle-testing technique to determine your optimal foods and how much of them to eat, it's important to remember to enjoy your meals. Food is your first friend, so why not consume it with joy and intention and make your dining experiences enjoyable and satisfying?

Think about the best meal you ever had. You likely remember more about it than just the food. What made that meal special or has made other memorable meals special for you? Almost everyone I have asked this question of replied that it was a meal eaten with loved ones or good friends, either home-cooked or at a special place. Not one person has mentioned calorie count, that they checked labels, or that they regretted that the food they ate was "bad" for them.

Eat Mindfully

A crust eaten in peace is better than a banquet partaken in anxiety.
– Aesop

If you have ever tried to communicate with someone who was checking their email, taking phone calls, or staring out the window, it probably hurt your feelings and made you feel taken for granted. Treating your food this way by not being mentally present, or mindful, while you eat can hurt your body, just as lack of attentiveness can destroy a relationship. Eating with distractions makes you eat faster, snack more, and disconnect from feeling full. You don't even remember what you have eaten throughout the day, known as "eating amnesia," which can result in eating a big meal not long after having already eaten one, or unconsciously snacking for hours on end. Twenty-four clinical studies performed by the American Journal of Clinical Nutrition showed that "attentive eating is likely to influence food intake, and incorporation of attentive-eating principles into interventions provides a novel approach to aid weight loss and maintenance without the need for conscious calorie counting." (https://www.ncbi.nlm.nih.gov/pmc/articles/PMC3607652)

Stop grabbing and gobbling meals on the go and eating in your car. Stop eating out of the refrigerator and grabbing food out of a box in your cupboard. Stop standing in the kitchen eating over the counter or eating in front of the TV. Put your food on a plate and take your plate to the table and sit down.

Make your meals *intentional.* If you are too busy to stop eating on the run, then you are too busy! Make the time to stop and sit when you eat.

This is easier for small families to do than large ones, yet it is a goal to strive for. Foster peace and calm in your home before and at meals. Watching the chaos and stress on the TV news while eating is really bad for your digestion!

Break Bread Together

Eating with others has a cascade of healthy benefits. Eating socially helps us feel happier and more satisfied with life. We feel more supported and connected. Think about friends and acquaintances you meet when you go out to events or to a restaurant; this interaction creates connection and social bonding in your community. A simple evening meal with others can create closeness, laughter, reminiscing, and satisfaction with life.

A research survey in the UK tested whether eating with others provided social or individual benefits and concluded that the causal direction runs from eating together to bondedness rather than the other way around. It is eating together that creates the bonding we feel at mealtime. (https://link.springer.com/article/10.1007/s40750-017-0061-4)

I came from a family where gravy is considered a beverage.
– Erma Bombeck

The family meal was a normal daily ritual in homes for generations. Over the past few decades the picture of the family sitting around the table chatting and communing together over a home-cooked meal has lost its focus.

It's a real balancing act for children with busy schedules and even busier parents to gather around the table at the same time. Many families seem more like a circus act trying to juggle all the activities. It is a grab-some-grub-and-go scenario too much of the time.

A number of studies showed that children who regularly ate dinner with their families were less likely to get involved in drugs and alcohol, than those who did not. They also tended to get better grades, exhibited less stress, and ate better. A study by the Columbia Center showed that compared with teenagers who ate five or more family dinners a week, those who ate two or fewer family dinners a week were three times as likely to try marijuana, two-and-a-half times as likely to smoke cigarettes, and one-and-a-half times as likely to try alcohol.

It wasn't long ago when my three boys were playing baseball in the spring and were on different teams, practicing and playing their games miles apart and at different times, and each had three weekly practices at different times and locations. And that was just baseball; there were scout meetings, school events, clubs, work schedules, a daughter involved in a lot of activities, and... well, if you have children, you know, don't you? We ate a lot of hurriedly made tuna sandwiches during the week, though we ate them together. I planned ahead and made special meals on Sundays and non-baseball nights.

Be flexible, but make family meals a priority. It's worth it to grow deep family ties and add more enjoyment to your meals. You might find that weekend breakfasts or lunches are the best times to eat together. The time of the meal isn't as important as gathering everyone around the table.

Turn your television off, put mail and reading material away, and turn your phones and computers off. Clear off any stuff that has collected on your table. Involve the family in setting the table and preparing the meal, or just keeping the cook company in the kitchen while they are doing so. Keep conversation on a positive note. Take heavy or stressful subjects that need to be discussed elsewhere, away from the table.

Zen and the Art of Cooking is a beautiful book by Jon Sandifer. It's about drawing on Eastern principles of *feng shui* and using the elements of energy in our relationships with food and cooking. Sandifer wrote that cooking, preparing, and serving a meal can be like a meditation:

If you value devoting some time every day to meditation or self-reflection, then you can save time by including cooking as part of your spiritual practice. Without the distractions of the TV, radio, or telephone, you have the opportunity to reflect on who you are cooking for, and what kind of chi (good energy) you would like to energize the food with. You can even visualize the outcome of the meal.

Make family meals a habit. Create your own traditions around preparing and eating food to love, honor, and nourish yourself and others.

A Family of One

A family is not any particular number of people. It can be the traditional parents and kids, any combination thereof plus extended family members and friends, or even just one person. It makes no difference who is at the table; you can still be considered a family.

Author and design educator Tim Gunn claimed, "There's nothing I like better than going to my apartment, closing the door, cooking my little dinner for one and just tuning out. My apartment really is my haven. It's a nest where I go to heal." If you are a family of one, it is just as important to honor yourself at mealtime, as it is for a couple or a larger family group. Don't neglect good eating habits just because you're alone. It can feel uncomfortable to sit by yourself at your table if you have not been doing this, and it might feel like it doesn't matter, but it's no less important than it is when you live with a tribe.

Set yourself a nice place at your table and *be* with yourself. Soft music is nice. Be present with your thoughts and enjoy your food. Think about the taste and texture, and chew slowly. Think pleasant thoughts. Light a candle and watch it flicker as you eat. This can help you focus and reduces stress. Do nothing else but eat. Practice enjoying this time with yourself and your food. This can be a very delightful and nurturing experience every day.

DAEO – Digest, Assimilate, Eliminate, and all Other

"Day-O, Day-ay-ay-O, Daylight come and me wan' go home!" Do you remember those lyrics from "The Banana Boat Song" belted out by Harry Belafonte? It became one of his signature songs in the '50s. When I was designing a digestion energy technique that would be easy for my clients to remember and fun to do, the acronym D.A.E.O. popped into my mind. I suddenly heard Harry belt out "Day-O, Day-ay-ay-O!" complete with calypso beat and bongo drums! It stands for Digest, Assimilate, Eliminate, and all Other.

I described these processes very simply in chapter 9. Your body, if healthy, processes your food naturally as you eat it. Yet the top-selling over-the-counter drugs on the market are digestive aids! Heartburn, nausea, gas, constipation, diarrhea, and digestion problems are epidemic. There are a lot of guts out there struggling. We need help with digestion!

In addition to the Gut Flush you can use my DAEO technique to balance your body's digestion. Here are the descriptions of the elements:

Digest: break down by chewing, including the breakdown process of enzymes and chemical actions in the gut

Assimilate: absorb and integrate digested food

Eliminate: completely remove what is not needed

All **Other**: balance any "other" part of digestion. There is still much that is unknown and being discovered about our bodies, and adding "other," as I do for all my energy techniques, simply includes anything else, known or unknown.

Muscle-Testing for DAEO

How is your Day-ay-ay-O? Test how well you are digesting, assimilating, and eliminating your food. Jot down your answers on a piece of paper. Ask:

- How well am I digesting food on a scale of 0 to 10? 0? 1? 2? [etc.]
- How well am I assimilating food on a scale of 0 to 10? 0? 1? 2? [etc.]

- How well am I eliminating on a scale of 0 to 10? 0? 1? 2? [etc.]
- How well are my "other" digestive functions on a scale of 0 to 10? 0? 1? 2? [etc.]

The answers to your DAEO muscle-testing might have surprised you. You can balance your digestion by sending an intention message via your governing meridian, as in the energy techniques I described above. The message flashes to all parts of your body, telling it to get to work, come into balance, and fulfill your command.

Energy-Balancing for DAEO

Swipe the top of your head from front to back with a magnet, the palm of your hand, or your fingertips while saying or thinking each of the DAEO elements three times, taking a nice deep breath in between:

- Digest
- Assimilate
- Eliminate
- All Other

(If you are doing this for another person, swipe from the top of their head down their back.)

Now go back to "Muscle-Testing for DAEO" above and ask the questions again to retest your ratings. Write down your new ratings, as they probably will have increased. You can do this exercise on a daily basis.

Bless Your Food

It has been proven scientifically that prayer changes frequencies, and food is a frequency. Expressing gratitude, giving thanks, and blessing food is an ancient energy technique. Prayer and gratitude may be the most important and profound energy techniques of all when it comes to intentional eating.

Gratitude shows you that the grass beneath your feet is greener than you think.
– Dr. Robert Holden

Ancient peoples danced together in celebration when preparing food, blessed the cooking pots and the cooks, and kissed the plates the food was served on. This actually sounds like my house when we get together, right down to loving our dishes. When you bless your food, it promotes mindfulness: calmly focusing on the present moment; drawing your attention to taste, texture, and flavor; and bringing forth more satisfaction and enjoyment. It brings a peaceful, happy feeling to the table, enhancing readiness for, eating as well as creating a communing experience with your meal.

I read a story of a woman who sat down at her table to eat a Twinkie and drink a glass of milk. She usually prayed over her food but as she looked at the Twinkie she said to herself, "Well, this isn't very nutritious." Immediately the thought popped into her mind, "It could be!" She stopped and offered a quick prayer.

Dr. Masaru Emoto believed that water could react to positive thoughts and words, and that polluted water could be cleaned through prayer and positive visualization. He published volumes of experimental work entitled *Messages from Water*. Emoto introduced different vibrations into water. He froze the water and captured pictures of the frozen water crystals. Many of his photos were of beautiful water *crystals* after playing good music and offering gratitude and prayers to the water.

I did an experiment with my kids when they were young, at about the time the knowledge was circulating that plants respond to love and good music. We soaked a bunch of mung bean seeds in water, divided the seeds into two equal groups, and planted them in two paper cups. On cup A we wrote "good" words like "I love you" and "Gratitude," and the kids drew things like hearts and smiley faces. On cup B we wrote "bad" words like "I hate you" and "You are bad," and the kids drew frowny faces and garbage, and one of the boys drew the worst thing he could think of: a pile of dog poop. If you have boys, I know you totally understand this!

Each cup received the same water and sunlight. Every day we said loving words or did loving things to cup A, including blessing it; and said mean things and scorned cup B. The results were noticeable. The blessed cup A seeds sprouted, grew quickly, and leafed out. Only about half the seeds in cup B sprouted, and the ones that did produced short, scrawny plants. Some mold showed up in the dirt.

This made an impact on my kids. In fact, some of my grandkids have used this experiment as science fair projects with very similar results.

In our family we have passed along the tradition and habit of giving thanks for the food we eat. It is very special to see a two-year-old baby fold her arms and bow her head as she utters a few words in her baby language before she eats.

> *Give me good digestion, Lord,*
> *And also something to digest;*
> *but where and how that something comes*
> *I leave to Thee, who knoweth best.*
> *– Mary Webb*

When you take a moment to express gratitude and bless your food before you eat it, the frequency of that food changes for the better. Your prayer can be a simple blessing of any kind that you have learned. You don't have to be Christian. You don't have to be Buddhist. Give thanks in your own way.

On his travels through fifty-two countries and four continents as a young man, author Jon Sandifer noticed:

The factor common to all the cultures where I was a guest was that the meal began with some form of appreciation or grace. It was usually nothing elaborate, but at least a few moments were taken either to thank the cook, or thank God for the food, or to wish good health on the people who were about to eat it.

If you are not used to doing this and would like to begin, start by speaking kindly, as you would to a best friend: "Thank you. Please be good for me." Focus love and gratitude on the food for a moment. It can be that brief and simple. When giving thanks to the Creator of food I also like to thank the food and add the DAEO – "Please digest, assimilate, eliminate and all other" – to my prayer.

It is not always possible to eat perfectly, even when you use the Food Codes method and all the muscle-testing tools in this book. Don't worry. Just do the best you can. Intention is everything. My motto is "Do your best and bless the rest." It works!

Food Is a Love Note from God

When you eat, you feed your soul as well as your body. Your diet impacts your spirit as well as your physical being.

> *Not only are we affected by the environment in which food is grown, we are also affected by the consciousness of the people who prepare our food. Marcel Vogel has shown that water infused with the thought form of Love has a different taste and a different subtle vibration. As we eat blessed food, we eat our blessings on this subtle level. We are interacting with food on subtle energy levels as well as on the material level of assimilation.*
> *– Rabbi Gabriel Cousens*

Here's a quick summary of the Food Codes method:

- Use muscle-testing and the Food Codes Food List at TheFoodCodes.com/lists to determine the ranking of each of the foods and beverages listed.
- Consume foods that test the highest. The higher the ranking, the more your body needs that food for optimal health.
- Eliminate or reduce eating foods rated low for the length of time that muscle-testing rates them as such.

- Enjoy your meals! Use the recipes in the next section to create your best meals. Be sure to follow the tips for making your meals pleasurable.
- Bless your food.
- Use the "Energy-Balancing for DAEO" technique.
- Use muscle-testing to know when you are hungry, and while you are eating to know when you are full. Stop eating when your body tells you to.
- When dining out select foods from your Food Codes plan or discreetly test menu items before ordering.
- Retest your Food Codes when the seasons change and when you experience a change in your life or lifestyle. If your intuition tells you a change is needed, retest to find what foods your body needs that day.
- Breathe, drink plenty of pure water, get some sunshine, and move your body in the ways it wants to.
- Do the 30-Second Gut Flush each morning and night.
- Revel in the additional energy, health, and wellness you experience in your marvelous body and the beautiful relationship you have with your best friend, food!

It is my deepest wish that you use the Food Codes and discover how easy it is to know what's best for you to eat. Trust your inner knower and your ability to use muscle-testing to access that inner knowledge.

Cooking and Recipes

CHAPTER 11
Reconnecting with Food

We have become disconnected from our food. Many children and a lot of adults don't know where food actually comes from. To get to our major food source we drive to a clean grocery store where the smell of freshly baked food is in the air. We choose our foods from a shelf or a refrigerated cooler as we listen to soothing music. Then we return home and shelve our groceries.

The average child might not know that a French fry is made from a potato grown underground in the dirt, or that an egg comes from the other end of a chicken. I know a child who stopped eating eggs for a long time when she discovered this shocking fact.

We can't all grow potatoes or raise chickens, yet we can reconnect with food in wonderful ways. One way is to buy whole foods like fresh vegetables, fruits, grains, meats, fish, and herbs. You don't have to scan a label; you can see right away that a tomato is a tomato. Reconnecting with food means preparing at least some of your meals from whole foods.

Another way to reconnect with food is to visit your local farmers' market. You will find fresh vegetables and fruits that may have been picked only hours ago; carrots with some dirt still clinging to them; freshly laid, free-range chicken eggs; and living herbs and plants. Take your kids or grandkids for a fun time. It's the easiest way to eat locally and seasonally. Ask the growers questions and learn about their produce from them. You might find a rainbow of different colored beets, carrots, and chard ready to go home in your bag, or things you've never heard of eating such as zucchini blossoms. They are delicious and can be prepared in several ways.

I count on my local farmers' market for shopping in season and buying foods in bulk for canning and preserving for the winter. I buy locally grown organic tomatoes by the case to make salsa and sauces. I buy twenty-pound bags of baby cucumbers and heads of fresh green dill weed and garlic to make the best kosher dill pickles ever. We eat these year-round, and I use them to make my famous (to family and friends anyway) Dill Pickle Potato Salad. I buy extra jars of freshly harvested local honey to store and to give as gifts.

Fall harvest time is a family get-together time at my house. It is a tradition of preserving healthy food that has been passed from my grandmothers and mother to me, and I am passing the healthy knowledge and tradition forward to my family, friends, those in my classes, and now you!

Reconnecting Communities through Local Food

A grassroots movement is spreading to reconnect individuals, communities, schools, and health care institutions to their local food growers, farmers, and ranchers. My son Jonathan is involved on the forefront of this movement in his community as executive chef of Livingston HealthCare hospital and Café

Fresh, located in beautiful Livingston, Montana. This health care facility is setting an example for other such institutions to model. Believe me when I tell you that this is one hospital that does not serve "hospital food"!

The folks at Livingston HealthCare believe that good food and healthy eating is key to healing their patients. With health care costs, chronic disease and obesity on the rise, they decided that health care providers need to find ways to increase health education and disease prevention in their community. They do this by providing healthy food and modeling healthy food choices through Café Fresh.

The goal of Livingston HealthCare is to promote health and wellness among patients and staff, so the hospital opened its doors to the community with a new state-of-the-art restaurant branded Café Fresh. Its design is unique in the hospital setting. The idea is that "people eat with their eyes," therefore most of the food choices offered at Café Fresh are on display at mealtimes. Foods are prepared from local, seasonal, fresh foods including locally raised and free-range meats like grass-fed beef and poultry; fruits; and vegetables. You will find huge stock pots of rich, nutritious, healthy broth slowly simmering in the Café Fresh kitchen as a healthy base for dishes, and weekly menus you would expect to find at only fine-dining restaurants. It's definitely not hospital food.

The result of this forward thinking in health care has been a big success, expanding customer taste palates for a variety of high-quality, healthy, fresh foods, including ethnic foods, and modeling positive eating habits. This earned Livingston HealthCare's Café Fresh the award for the Top Farm to

Healthcare Institution in The Nation for 2017. The successful program has increased revenue benefits for the community and Montana by supporting local growers and local job creation.

The success of this program inspired Livingston area schools and other hospitals across the state to model it. Jonathan leant his hand with volunteer cooking for the local food bank. He headed a free community course teaching chef skills, so people could get better jobs to support their families.

Reconnecting with our best friend, food, starts with each one of us. And as we reconnect, this energy sends out far-reaching ripples into our communities and beyond.

Ban Excuses for Not Cooking

"People don't cook these days" is something I hear a lot. On the other hand, I see top-rated TV shows about cooking, millions subscribing to cooking magazines and cooking blogs, and floods of food pictures on social media sites. This boils down to two things in my mind: it is true that we eat with our eyes; and yes, some people do cook.

I define the word *cooking* as not necessarily subjecting food to heat, but the art or craft of preparing food for consumption. A survey taken by the Bosch kitchen appliance company was profiled in a 2011 Marketwire article called "What's Keeping Americans out of Their Kitchens? National Survey Reveals the Top Excuses for Not Cooking." Over 50 percent of Americans said they didn't cook because their spouse or partner did all the cooking. 25 percent said they didn't want to clean up the mess. And 21 percent replied they didn't have time. In further questions 66 percent said that the most time-consuming household chore is shopping, and 28 percent of respondents admitted that they just plain didn't know how to cook. (http://www.marketwired.com/press-release/whats-keeping-americans-out-their-kitchens-national-survey-reveals-top-excuses-not-1558601.htm)

Cooking can now be completely outsourced. You never have to shop to stock your kitchen or even turn on your oven. You don't even have to leave your house. You can buy premade packaged meals that are shipped right to your door no matter where you live.

But I believe food preparation should be one of the rituals *you* perform to care for yourself. Think of the daily rituals you have learned to do automatically like bathing, fixing your hair, brushing your teeth, cleaning your ears, shaving, and putting on your makeup. They became automatic only after you learned how to do them. It's the same for preparing food; it can become an easy daily ritual.

Preparing your own food and feeding yourself is a personal and intimate act of self-care. Learning the simple basics and making a habit of it can be as essential to your well-being as it was to learn how to brush your teeth. Anyone with the desire can learn the basics, and preparing good foods for yourself and your family can become an automatic and easy self-care ritual.

I have lots of older siblings, and as they started to leave the house, I went from cooking once a week to twice, three times, and so on. After a while, it was just like making the bed.
— Hugh Jackman

My husband and I were in the 50 percent of Americans for whom one spouse did all the cooking. Before I met Bruce his grocery list was Pepsi, gummy bears, salted nut rolls, and chips. He ate his meals out.

The first time I was at his house it was huckleberry season and I decided to make a pie from fresh-picked huckleberries. I asked him where items like flour and shortening were in his kitchen and he just looked at me blankly and said, "I don't know. I have never opened the cupboards." He had lived there for five years!

So I prepare the majority of our meals, yet Bruce has taken it upon himself in the last couple of years to learn some cooking. He makes a great egg omelet that he is quite proud of.

Do you make excuses for not cooking, feel there are drawbacks to preparing food for yourself and your family, or have any hang-ups about cooking? Maybe you just hate it, fear learning about it, or feel you really don't have the time. Perhaps you used to cook for your family but no longer bother to cook for yourself. Try the easy ten-minute meditation and clearing exercise below to clear any mental blocks you discover.

Energy-Balancing Exercise for Happy Cooking

Have paper and pen ready to write down the impressions that come to your mind.

Step 1: Discover the block.

a. Sit comfortably and relax.

b. Take a few deep breaths and relax even more as you notice your breathing. Let your shoulders drop and your tummy soften. Close your eyes if that helps you relax more.

c. Ask, "Do I have a block associated with cooking?" If yes, write down as many as come to mind. Examples of what may come up are "I'm not good at it," "I don't know how," "There's not enough time," and "I'm too busy."

d. Choose the block that feels the strongest and move to step 2. If no block revealed itself, move to step 2 using "I have a block to cooking" as your block.

Step 2: Clear the block.

a. Muscle-test for how strong the block feels on a scale of 0 to 10, and write down the number.

b. Use a magnet, the palm of your hand, or your fingertips to swipe the top of your head from front to back while saying or thinking, "I release [name of block]. (If you are doing this for another person, swipe down their back.) Do this two more times.

c. Take a nice deep breath.

d. Again, muscle-test for how strong the block feels on a scale of 0 to 10, and write down the number.

e. If the block has cleared, you can do this again with another block. If the block still rates high, continue clearing and rechecking until you feel like the block has diminished or released.

Many people find that they feel neutral about the block after doing this exercise. Neutral is good; it means the negative vibration has released. They also note that naming their block now feels silly or even ridiculous. You can do this exercise over and over with other thoughts or problems you have regarding your relationship to preparing food and cooking.

While I was writing this chapter, I did this exercise myself. I love to cook, and I cook a lot. I would not have thought I had any blocks to cooking. I stopped typing for a minute and took a deep breath and asked myself, "Do I have any blocks to cooking?" A voice entered my mind: "I'm too busy!" It was my mother's voice and I could see myself standing at the stove in her kitchen when I was thirteen years old. She was telling me that she had gotten a job and cooking dinner every day was now up to me. I had five younger siblings, and she expected dinner to be ready when she and my dad got home from work. Take-out food was not an option in those days. I released "I am too busy" by doing Step 2 of the "Energy-Balancing Exercise for Happy Cooking.".

What popped up for me next was "I *never* get to have fun." Life changed when my mom started working outside our home. I kept watch over my wild little brothers and made sure dinner was on the table by 5:30 when mom and dad got home. That was just the way it was. When I started to release "I *never* get to have any fun," a heavy feeling of sadness welled up like a weight on my chest. As I continued, the weight slowly lifted. I had to repeat the exercise three times to completely release it. I have no doubt that releasing "I *never* get to have any fun," which showed up as a block to cooking, will change other aspects of my life so I can be free to have more fun!

My family members were good sports about my morphing cooking skills. I learned about the importance of timing when

I made a "breakfast for dinner" meal of hash brown potatoes, bacon, and fried eggs: don't make the eggs first! A stack of fried eggs sitting for an hour turns to cold rubber.

Eating Well

> *For is there any practice less selfish, any labor less alienated, any time less wasted, than preparing something delicious and nourishing for people you love?*
> *– Michael Pollan*

Free yourself from the restrictions of recipes forever and enjoy stress-free cooking! The best chefs employ a few basic ratios of ingredients and five basic flavors to create any dish or meal. Learning this concept is like knowing how to cook all recipes.

Break free from having to eat traditional meals. You might have soup or a salad for breakfast, or not be hungry until brunchtime. You don't need to have advanced cooking skills to feed yourself with nourishing foods, just a desire to nourish your body.

In this section you will find ideas about how to put basic foods together to eat well. You will learn how to make simple meals from simple foods, cooking from scratch without a script. Cooking will become a part of your daily ritual that is so fulfilling you won't remember not knowing how to do it.

> *I was 32 when I started cooking; up until then, I just ate.*
> *– Julia Child*

Mark Bittman taught *How to Cook Everything* in his book by that name. Cooking at its heart is simple and straightforward.

He said that you work through a few basic tasks to get from point A to point B, moving toward your goal to eat. He believes that home cooking is important because it's satisfying, saves money, and produces nutritious food, and is time well spent and very rewarding.

Cooking leads to family meals. Family meals stimulate conversation, communication, and love. It's a fact.
– Mark Bittman

We express ourselves through everything we do. Cooking is a form of self-expression, so add a little love and feel good when you cook. Using your Food Codes plan, put together meals with the foods that test the best for you. Doing this with your own flair of self-expression is rewarding, healthy, and saves money and time. Yes, time! You can cook your own healthy meal in less time than it takes the pizza delivery guy to find your house.

People who love to eat are always the best people.
– Julia Child

CHAPTER 12

Getting Ready to Cook

How to Use the Recipes

The Food Codes Food List is a list of ordinary whole foods that are widely available. At the bottom of each category you can add any "other" food that you would like to test and add. Use your top foods to cook with and of course avoid the others as much as possible.

Let's say you are making vegetable soup and you have selected the main ingredients from several of your top vegetables, but onions test low for you and you love the flavor of onions. Go ahead and add a little onion; a little won't make a big difference.

How to Use the Recipe Templates

Using the recipe templates is simply using approximate measurements with a variety of ingredients. Keep your best foods on hand to be ready to make a recipe at any time.

To create your own recipe, first think about what you would like to eat in general terms, like soup for instance. Then decide whether your taste buds are hungry for something spicy, like chicken tortilla soup, or a comfort food, like chicken noodle soup. These two soups are very similar, yet differ dramatically due to only a couple of ingredients. Thinking in general terms like this teaches you how to cook by instinct. You won't have to take the time to search for a recipe and then run to the store to get the odd ingredient that you don't have.

Each recipe is designed as a template from which to build your own individual recipe using your best foods. The templates can be used in many ways to make endless combinations. Let this be a new and fun experience!

You might find that you can reconstruct some of your own favorite recipes by switching out a couple of ingredients that are not on your Food Codes plan. People who invent recipes just use what they have on hand at the time.

If this sounds overwhelming, go back to the "Energy-Balancing for Happy Cooking" exercise above and release that overwhelm or whatever it is that's blocking you from creating your own healthy meals. Following your intuitive guidance to cooking and eating really can become a simple, fun and easy lifestyle.

In the following chapters you will find suggestions for how to use your best foods with each template. I show you some actual Food Codes plans from people who use the Food Codes and examples of recipes that were created using them. I give you ideas for other possibilities in order to help you create interesting and satisfying dishes without having to rely on traditional recipes.

How a food is prepared can make a difference in its health value as well as taste. Should it be eaten raw, cooked, sprouted, or juiced? You can ask any of these questions using the muscle-testing technique below. Test foods in your Food Codes plan to see if the way they are prepared makes a difference. When preparing beans, grains, seeds, and nuts, the value ratings can change quite a bit depending on how they are prepared. For example, pinto beans out of a can might not be a best food for you; however, if you test the value of cooking pinto beans yourself, and cooking them in certain ways, they might test as one of your better foods. The reasons for this are explained in the following sections.

Muscle-Testing for Food Preparation

Some of the questions below won't apply to all foods; just test foods and cooking methods that apply. Test for yes or no, or go a step further and test the value on a scale of 0 to 10. Insert the name of the food where there are blanks.

- Does the way ___ is/are prepared make a difference for me? (If no, you don't need to test any further.)
- Is/are ___ best for me raw?
- Is/are ___ best for me cooked?
- Is/are ___ best for me juiced?
- Is/are ___ best for me canned?

You might find that soaking (or soaking and sprouting) beans and grains raises the value of the food for you. Use the questions below with beans, lentils, grains, seeds, and nuts.

- Does the way ___ is/are prepared make a difference for me? (If no, you don't need to test any further.)
- Is/are ___ best for me canned?

- Is/are ____ best for me home-cooked?
- Is/are ____ best for me soaked?
- Is/are ____ best for me soaked and sprouted?

Basic Cooking Methods

Cooking can be a balancing act. Cook times and temperatures vary with the cooking method used and the altitude where you live. The recipe templates in this book are general suggestions, and different types of applied heat, steam, and pressure have a wide variety of effects on cooking foods.

Blanch: Food is dropped carefully in boiling water to scald; removed after a brief, timed interval; then carefully plunged into iced water or placed under cold running water to release heat and stop the cooking process. Used for fruits, especially tomatoes, to release and remove the skins. Partially cooks soft vegetables to be eaten tender-crisp. Softens tough greens like kale, collards, and mustard greens. Prepares vegetables for freezing.

Sauté (or Stir-Fry): From a French word meaning "to jump," sauté means to cook quickly. Food is placed in a hot pan on medium-high heat, with a small amount of fat, and tossed while cooking. Simply use a spatula and keep turning the food quickly until just cooked. Used for vegetables and meats.

Steam: Using moist heat to cook food. Use a two-part steamer pot with a lid (any pot with a steamer tray works). Add water to the bottom part of the pot, place the food in the steamer basket above the water, and put the lid on. Bring the pot to a slow boil while steam cooks the food. Foods that steam quickly such as spinach and other greens should be added after the water comes to a boil so they don't get soggy. Used for vegetables, fish, seafood, meats, and other foods.

Boil: Immerse food in water or liquid and bring to a boil. Turn the heat down just enough to keep the water boiling and cook until done. Used for vegetables, eggs, rice, meats, sauces, and soups.

Parboil: Immerse food in water and cook about half-way or to the desired doneness, then continue cooking using another method. Hard vegetables can be parboiled first to quicken cooking time, like before grilling or putting into a stir-fry or casserole. Used for artichokes, potatoes, Brussels sprouts, and other vegetables.

Bake: Cooking in dry heat in the oven, covered or uncovered. Used for all kinds of foods.

Roast: Cooking in dry heat in the oven, uncovered on a pan or cooking tray. Brings out the liquids and browns the food. Used for vegetables and meats.

Grill: Dry-heat cooking with hot heat or flame from below, such as on a barbeque grill. Used for vegetables, meats, fish, and many other foods.

Broil: Heat applied from just above the food, as in your oven broiler. Used to quickly brown vegetables, meats, and fish.

Slow Cooker/Crockpot: An electric countertop appliance used for unattended cooking to cook foods slowly for hours. Used for soups, stews, vegetables, desserts, and many other dishes.

Pressure Cooker: Cooks food four times faster than boiling and baking. A low level of water or other cooking liquid is put in the pot with the food and the pot is sealed shut. The trapped steam increases the pressure in the pot and allows the temperature to rise higher than in boiling, resulting in cooking the food faster. It saves nutrients, energy, and time. Stove-top or electric pressure-cooking is as safe as any other method of cooking. Used for everything from "baked" potatoes to grains, roasts, ribs, chicken, beans, vegetables, soups, eggs, bone broth, breads, and much more. A pressure cooker is a kitchen essential if you want to speed up the cook time for fast, nutritious meals. It can also be used for canning. My pressure cookers are my absolute best friends in the kitchen. I have both stove-top and electric pressure cookers.

Microwave: Heats foods very quickly. Microwaves cause water molecules in food to vibrate, producing heat that cooks the food. Used for all foods.

Five Essential Flavors – The Foundation for Seasoning Foods

Don't settle for bland food! Flavor matters! Why eat food that doesn't taste good, even if it's the best thing for you? The four basic types of flavor are salt, acid, fat, and sweet, and all other flavors available from spices and other sources I lump into the fifth flavor category. You can create a variety of delicious flavors through the seasonings you use.

When seasoning food, a little dab'll do ya most of the time. My daughter Natalie, who is now a professional pastry chef, learned this the hard way when she cooked spaghetti as a surprise dinner for our family. She was about thirteen years old at the time. She poked through the spice cabinet and dumped the spices into her spaghetti sauce that she said "looked" like they would go into spaghetti sauce. It looked and smelled delicious, but everyone stopped short with the first couple of chews. Natalie looked up and said, "I think I added too much of something." She started listing off spices she used, continuing, "And I put in cloves because they were brown and looked like they would go with the sauce." She had added *a lot* of cloves! Cloves, one of the most bitter, pungent flavors of the spice world, had taken over Natalie's spaghetti sauce.

Every part of the world has its own notes of flavor and variety of seasonings with signature flavors, like Asian, Italian, and Indian, yet every flavor starts with the basic essentials of salt, acid, fat, and/or sweet. The key is to taste as you prepare, adjusting the flavor as you cook, and taste it again before serving to see if it needs something more. That doesn't mean to eat a meal as you're cooking! A little taste will tell you what it needs. Coming to a meal hungry enhances your enjoyment of the food.

Salt: Salt brings out natural flavors, preserves color, preserves food, and controls the dominance of harmful bacteria in fermented foods. It can draw moisture out of vegetables to soften them faster and improves tenderness in meats. Many foods are rich with natural salt, such as celery and seaweed. Sea salt is less refined than table salt, plays a part in good health, and enhances flavor. Salt a little at first. You need less sea salt than table salt. If you add too much salt, expand your recipe to a double batch.

Acid: Many "acid" or acidic foods are alkalinizing when eaten (the opposite of acidic on the pH scale), like tomatoes, tomato sauce, citrus fruit, and apple cider vinegar. "Acid" does not mean that these foods are acidic to the body. Honey, mustard, olive oil, and fermented dairy products lean toward being acidic, yet tend to be alkalinizing.

Acids come in a wide variety of flavors. Vinegars range from very tart, like apple cider vinegar; to sweet, like balsamic vinegar. A squeeze of a lemon, lime, or other citrus fruit, or a dash of vinegar, can enhance flavor as well as digestion.

Acid foods affect the color, texture, and flavor of food and can cause chemical reactions when used as leavening agents, such as when combining baking soda and vinegar to help a quick bread rise when baking. Acidic foods like fermented sauerkraut, sour cream, yogurt, natural cheese, pickles, tomatoes, and hot sauce can complement the flavors of many dishes. A touch of acid, like a dash of vinegar, makes flavors sparkle.

Fat: Fat, plain and simple, makes food taste good. The aromatic and flavor components of foods are mostly fat-soluble, not water soluble. Fat feels good in your mouth and can even make a flavor last longer in your mouth. Good "mouth feel" is one of the main things that manufacturers create for their food products. Fat helps carry flavor in a recipe, enriches nutrition, and facilitates cooking many foods, such as keeping food from sticking to the pan. Research the information on "good" fats if you have been raised to think fat is bad for you. It's not!

The wide variety of flavors in fats bring about wonderful culinary combinations. Fat flavors relate to many cuisines, like sesame oil in Asian food, fragrant olive oil in Italian food, and of course butter in French dishes. Some fats are delicate and fare better in the heat of cooking than others. Oils can be infused with herbs for flavor and be sprinkled over cooked food for a nutritious drizzle of flavor. Fat is derived from plants and animals. There are probably several that rate high for you – they are not all "bad" as some would have you think, and do not contribute to weight gain when used in moderation.

Fat is emulsified or broken down by bile salts in our bodies for proper digestion. Certain ingredients mixed together do the same thing. Whip eggs and oil together to make mayonnaise. Mustard mixed with oil and vinegar emulsifies to make a creamy dressing that will not separate.

Sweet: Sugar, like salt, is a natural flavor enhancer that adds to the flavor profile of a dish. Many foods are naturally sweet like fruits, dates, honey, real maple syrup, and molasses. Stevia is very popular as a sweetener; it's derived from an herb, but any type of stevia on your grocery store shelf is highly refined using added chemicals.

Sweeteners like honey are natural humectants, meaning they help foods like baked goods retain moisture and keep them from drying out. Sweeteners also aid in fermentation of foods. Some vegetables are sweet, like carrots, sweet potatoes, parsnips, fennel, beets, and peas. Balsamic vinegar is naturally sweet.

Keep in mind that the flavor of the sweetener affects the flavor and texture of foods. Experiment with natural sweeteners to get to know how they affect food on your Food Codes plan.

Other flavors: Spices provide a broad range of flavors to use in preparing food, and some flavors such as garlic and onion are common in many cuisines. As explained above, think of what you would like to eat and then think of flavors that would enhance that dish.

Bitter is a flavor that compliments many foods and does not get much mention. Many spices actually come from bitter foods such as ginger and mustard, and bitter flavor is found in many foods and herbs. Dark, leafy greens like kale; certain vegetables like Brussels sprouts; citrus peel; cocoa beans; and yerba mate, most commonly used to make yerba mate tea, are bitter foods.

Umami (oo-mah-mee), or savory flavor, has been described as meaty. A Japanese scientist, who experimented to find out what gives seaweed soup a rich, meaty flavor, discovered monosodium glutamate (MSG) through an extreme refining process. MSG has since been widely used to enhance flavor in food. We have specific taste receptors for umami. Umami foods include seaweed, soy sauce, parmesan cheese, fermented dairy products, mushrooms, tomatoes, and chocolate. Add bitter or umami flavors to sweet or spicy foods for palate-pleasers; for example, combine chocolate with sugar.

Spicy hot, also called spicy, is a flavor found in many cuisines. This flavor comes from peppers and seasonings. Just a bit perks up almost any dish you can imagine.

* * *

Eat your food slowly to really taste it and become more aware of food flavors. Feel in your mouth and on your tongue where you taste specific flavors. Experiment with combining flavors and see what turns your taste buds on.

Foundational Cooking Spices, Flavors, and Uses

Spice	Flavor qualities	Uses	Pairs with
Basil	sweet	poultry, vegetables, eggs, salads, wraps, dressings, sauces	garlic, oregano, rosemary, thyme
Bay leaves	bitter	meat, seafood, soups, beans, lentils, grains, broth/stock, vegetables, marinade	oregano, rosemary, thyme
Cayenne/ Chili pepper	spicy hot	meat, poultry, fish, soups, salads, beans, lentils, grains, marinade, sauces	cumin, cinnamon, paprika, garlic, oregano
Chives	sweet	poultry, fish, soups, sour cream, toppings, potato, vegetables, eggs	cayenne, garlic, paprika
Cinnamon	earthy, sweet	poultry, lamb, fruits, squash, sweet potato, breads, desserts, sauces	allspice, ginger, nutmeg, cloves, coriander
Coriander	earthy, peppery	poultry, beef, pork, fish, soups, beans, lentils, grains, curry, marinade	cumin, chili pepper, cinnamon

Spice	Flavor qualities	Uses	Pairs with
Cumin	earthy, smoky	poultry, beef, pork, fish, soups, beans, lentils, grains, curry, marinade, salsa	basil, oregano, garlic, turmeric, ginger, cinnamon, cayenne, chili pepper, paprika
Garlic	savory	poultry, beef, pork, fish, soups, beans, lentils, grains, curry, marinade, salsa	oregano, turmeric, cayenne, chili pepper, coriander, turmeric
Ginger	warm, sweet	poultry, beef, pork, carrot, squash, beet, sweet potato, rice, stir-fry, curry, sauces, marinade	coriander, garlic, nutmeg
Oregano	earthy	poultry, beef, pork, soups, beans, lentils, grains, marinade, salsa, tomato, vegetables	bay leaf, basil, garlic, cumin, chili pepper, rosemary, thyme

Spice	Flavor qualities	Uses	Pairs with
Paprika/ Sweet Pepper	sweet, warm	eggs, poultry, lamb, shellfish, cauliflower, broccoli, bell pepper, rice, soups, sauces, salad dressing	garlic, chili pepper, cumin, cinnamon
Rosemary	earthy	poultry, eggs, lamb, fish, potato, vegetables, marinade	bay leaf, basil, garlic, oregano, parsley, thyme
Thyme	earthy	poultry, beef, fish, pork, soups, beans, lentils, grains, marinade, sauces, tomato, vegetables	bay leaf, basil, garlic, oregano, rosemary
Turmeric	peppery, bitter	poultry, fish, cabbage, cauliflower, potato, garbanzo beans, lentils, curry, rice	garlic, ginger, cayenne, chili pepper, coriander, cumin

Aromatic Foods

An *aromatic* in the culinary world is a food that boosts the flavor or aroma of a dish. They are the secret weapons of top chefs and cooks. They include spices, herbs, vinegars, wine, citrus fruit, garlic, tomatoes, leeks, mushrooms, peppers, and parsnips, and can be combined in endless combinations.

"Aromatics" often refers to a simple, traditional mix of onion, celery, and carrot sautéed in fat. This combination has been used for centuries in every kind of cuisine. The French call it mirepoix (meer-pwa). Cooking in fat releases the deep flavors of the mix. It is used as a foundation for sautés, stir-frys, rice dishes, stocks, soups, stews, curries, and sauces. (See the mirepoix recipe in the "Sauces" section of the following chapter.)

More Flavors

Of course, I could not possibly include all the flavors used in cooking in the chart above. If you're curious about a spice or food you don't find above or in the Food Codes Food List, simply muscle-test it to find out if it's currently a good food for you.

CHAPTER 13
Recipes

Recipe Templates

Most ingredients and measurements in the following recipe templates can be changed according to taste and what ingredients muscle-test high for you. Use what you have on hand, and you can use more or less of each ingredient. Use the templates as guidelines. Refer to the appendices for converting various types of measurements.

Salads

My Grandma Violet was a wonderful cook. She cooked huge meals for the harvest crews on their farm in Idaho. My first memory of eating salad was at Grandma Violet's table when I was little. She would serve a plate of crisp iceberg lettuce cut into wedges, with nothing on it. We'd sprinkle a spoonful of sugar on top as we passed around her little desert-rose china sugar jar, and that was "salad." It was sweet, crunchy, and juicy, and I loved it. Grandma Violet put a little sugar in just about everything, and a lot of love, to enhance the flavor.

You can start your day with a fresh, bright salad for breakfast. After all, a green smoothie is really just a blended salad in a cup. This is a wonderful way to use vegetables and fruits from your Food Codes plan.

Salads can be concocted from anything from fresh greens to tubers, such as potatoes, and root vegetables, such as beets. Fruits, grains, and seeds make luscious salads that can be enjoyed at any meal, as a side dish or main course.

Quality ingredients are the key to true salad joy. Green salads are hydrating, contain up to 90 percent water, and are packed with nutrition and electrolytes. Experiment with fresh herbs and spices in your salads to expand your tastes. They have many health-promoting qualities. You only need half as much dried herbs if a recipe calls for fresh herbs.

Salad Greens, Flavors, and How to Use Them

Salad greens	Flavors	Qualities/Uses	Pairs with
Iceberg lettuce	mild, sweet	crisp and watery; serve chopped, shredded, in wedges, or with mixed greens and vegetables	heavy, creamy dressings; savory; ranch; blue cheese; chopped meat; poultry; croutons
Baby spring greens/ mesclun	mild, delicate	delicate mix of baby greens, lettuce, beet greens; makes a light side salad	light, sweet dressings; vinaigrettes

Salad greens	Flavors	Qualities/Uses	Pairs with
Spinach	mild to slightly bitter	small to medium leaves; serve with mixed greens, fruit, dried cranberries, and nuts	light, sweet dressings; light vinaigrettes
Leafy red or green lettuce	mild	large, frilly, delicate leaves that add volume and hold on to salad dressing; center rib adds a watery crunch	light, creamy dressings; balsamic vinaigrettes
Romaine lettuce	mild	center rib with leafy, watery leaves; traditional Caesar salad, multiple uses	light to heavy creamy dressings, Caesar dressing, vinaigrettes
Butter, Boston, and Bibb lettuce	mild, buttery	buttery flavor; creamy, crisp texture; use alone or with other mixed greens	light, creamy dressings; salty, crisp pancetta; bacon; light vinaigrette
Arugula	spicy, peppery	use with other greens to add contrast and a spark of flavor	simple vinaigrette to let the flavor shine through.

Salad greens	Flavors	Qualities/Uses	Pairs with
Watercress, Chicory, Radicchio, Endive	bitter and spicy	use with other greens to add contrast and interesting flavors	simple, light vinaigrette to let the flavor shine through
Red and green cabbage	sweet	sturdy and crunchy; shred for slaw; adds sweet flavor and crunch sprinkled on a lighter salad	heavy, creamy dressings; vinaigrettes
Chard, Mustard greens, Mature beet greens	strong, slightly bitter	Shred, chop finely, or blanch; cool in ice water; then chop. They're tough, so they add crunch to other greens or a warm sautéed salad.	acidic or vinaigrette dressing, chopped meat or poultry, nuts, citrus zest
Kale (any kind)	strong, slightly bitter	It's tough, so chop it and marinade in an acidic dressing overnight.	acidic or vinaigrette dressing

Green Salad Recipe Template

Use any combination of the freshest greens in any proportions you like, and voilà, you have a green salad.

Guidelines

1 head romaine, leafy, or iceberg lettuce is approximately 8 to 10 cups

1 pound of spinach is approximately 12 cups

1 serving of a side salad is 1 to 1 ½ cups

1 serving of salad as a main dish is 2 to 2 ½ cups

Directions

1. Remove outer leaves that are damaged or wilted. Separate the leaves from the stem; or to remove the core of an iceberg lettuce, smack the lettuce head, core down, sharply on a counter and twist out the core. Don't cut it out as it will turn brown.

2. Rinse to remove dirt and insects, then pat dry with a paper towel. Salad greens must be dry to hold the dressing. Using a salad spinner makes washing and drying very quick and easy, and you can store salad greens in the salad spinner bowl for later use.

3. Chop or tear the greens into bite-sized pieces. Tearing looks nicer and greens like lettuce won't brown at the edge as they do when cut with a knife.

A salad made with just greens, kept tightly sealed, lasts several days in the refrigerator if no dressing has been added. Serve with dressing of your choice.

Wedge Salad

Disregard any bad press about iceberg lettuce, especially if it's one of your top foods. Some say it is not worth eating as it is low in nutritional value. I disagree. It's a source of many nutrients as well as electrolyte-filled water for good hydration.

A classic wedge salad serving is one-fourth of a head of iceberg lettuce drizzled with a creamy dressing like blue cheese and sprinkled with various toppings. Tailor your toppings to fit your Food Codes plan. It's a super simple favorite any time of the year. Make it a meal by adding a lot of extra toppings such as diced apples, crumbled meat, other proteins such as beans or tofu, and vegetables.

Directions

Remove the outer leaves of an iceberg lettuce, rinse well under cold water, and pat dry with a paper towel. Do not remove the core as it holds the wedges together. Cut into four wedges from top to bottom and add toppings.

Topping Options

- Dried fruit: cranberries, raisins
- Fresh fruit: diced tomatoes, apples, berries
- Vegetables: any sliced, diced, shredded, chopped, pickled, or cooked beets, green onions, red or yellow onions, carrots, sweet peppers, roasted peppers, cucumbers, radishes, or any leftover vegetables you have around
- Nuts and seeds: whole, sliced, or chopped sesame, pumpkin, or sunflower seeds
- Hard-boiled eggs, sliced, wedged, or diced

- Meat, poultry, seafood: crumbled bacon, chicken, ham, turkey, beef, salmon, shrimp, crab
- Other proteins: beans, tofu, edamame
- Cheese: crumbled blue, feta, or any other dairy or non-dairy cheese
- Bread: croutons, bread crumbs
- Fresh herbs: basil, tarragon, cilantro
- Fresh-ground pepper and other spices

Salad Bar

My family loves a salad bar. It can kick off your meal or you can include extra food choices to pile on for a main meal. Create a salad bar to fit everyone's Food Codes plan by adding foods from each person's plan. Just set out one bowl of fresh greens prepared as in "Green Salad Recipe Template" above, bowls of options to add to the greens, and a variety of dressings. Use any of the items listed under "Topping Options" above, plus any of these that are good foods for those you're feeding:

- Dried fruit: dates, figs
- Fresh fruit: avocado, citrus slices, grapes, figs, pears, pineapple
- Legumes: any cooked beans, lentils, garbanzo beans
- Mushrooms: fresh or cooked
- Grains: any cooked grain
- Pasta
- Sprouts

Melon Salad Recipe Template

Ingredients

Sweet melon – about 8 cups cubed into bite-sized pieces

Greens – 1 or 2 cups

Sea salt – about 1 teaspoon

Vinaigrette dressing of your choice

Directions

Place melon in a large bowl, sprinkle greens on top, sprinkle with salt, drizzle dressing over the top to taste, and gently toss.

Other Possibilities

- Replace vinaigrette with fresh lime or lemon juice and olive oil.
- Add a dash of hot pepper sauce or ground chili pepper.
- Add very thinly sliced sweet onion.
- Add sliced Kalamata olives and feta cheese.
- Add fresh basil or mint leaves.
- Sprinkle with black sesame or poppy seeds.

Salad Dressings

Dressings have endless possibilities, and it's fun to play around and experiment with herb and spice combinations. Homemade dressings taste better and are fresher and healthier than anything you can buy, and they are super easy and inexpensive to make. You can whip up an easy dressing in five minutes. The ratios given below are for learning how to make dressings in general; they can be varied to your taste and desire.

Vinaigrette, the Queen of Dressings

The key to vinaigrette dressing is the ratio of 1 part vinegar to 3 parts oil. This is the gold standard. You can create a wide variety of dressings using different acids and different oils. If you don't use any fresh ingredients, like fresh herbs, you don't have to refrigerate it.

Directions

1. Combine 1 part vinegar with 3 parts oil in a bowl or jar.
2. Add salt, pepper, mustard, sugar, honey, or any flavoring you like.
3. Mix well. Use a blender to keep it emulsified longer.

Vinegar Options

- Apple cider vinegar
- Balsamic vinegar, dark or white
- Wine vinegar
- Lemon, lime, or orange juice

Oil Options

- Extra virgin olive oil
- Grapeseed
- Almond
- Avocado
- Sunflower
- Nut

Flavor Options

- Salt
- Pepper

- Small minced garlic clove
- 1/4 cup chopped basil, dill, or parsley
- 1 inch fresh ginger root, peeled and finely diced
- Basil
- Garlic powder or minced clove
- Shallot, minced
- Marjoram
- Oregano
- Onion, diced
- Ginger, fresh, chopped
- Prepared mustard such as stone-ground, hot, and Dijon
- 1 Tablespoon honey or another sweetener
- 2 to 4 Tablespoons Parmesan, blue, feta, or any other dairy or non-dairy cheese
- 2 or 3 mashed, oil-packed anchovies
- 1 Tablespoon or more fish sauce, which tames the vinegar flavor and adds another savory element
- 2 Tablespoons yogurt, sour cream, coconut cream, or canned coconut milk makes it into a creamy vinaigrette

My taste buds were in love with balsamic vinegar the first time we met. I put it on everything! My daughter Jennifer gave me a bottle of chocolate balsamic syrup – yes, chocolate and balsamic vinegar married in a rich sauce. It was amazing drizzled over ice cream and dessert. Another daughter, Whitney, introduced me to Modena white balsamic vinegar, which has become the darling of my kitchen. I drizzle it on foods to bring out a spark of brightness.

Balsamic Vinaigrette Recipe Template

Made with dark balsamic vinegar, this dressing is rich, dark, and smooth. Made with white balsamic vinegar it looks like liquid satin. Honey or maple syrup helps emulsify it.

Ingredients for 1 cup dressing

1/4 cup balsamic vinegar, dark or white

1 or 2 Tablespoons honey or real maple syrup

1/2 teaspoon granulated or powdered garlic or onion (optional)

1/4 teaspoon salt or to taste (optional)

1/4 teaspoon pepper (optional)

3/4 cup grapeseed oil

Directions

1. In a bowl combine balsamic vinegar, honey or syrup, and seasonings.
2. Stir to combine.
3. Quickly whisk mixture as you slowly drizzle in the oil. Or shake in a jar or combine in a blender.
4. Taste test and modify flavors if needed.

Ranch Dressing Recipe Template

Ingredients

3/4 cup plain yogurt

1 teaspoon dried or 3 teaspoons fresh dill weed

1/2 teaspoon powdered or granulated garlic or onion

1/4 teaspoon each of salt and pepper, or to taste

1/4 cup mild-tasting oil like almond, avocado, sunflower, or light olive oil

Directions

1. Using a small blender or food processor, blend yogurt, dill, garlic or onion, salt, and pepper.
2. Very slowly add the oil while blending so that it emulsifies.
3. Use immediately or store up to four days in the fridge.

Other Possibilities

- Substitute for yogurt: 3/4 cup Greek yogurt, sour cream, coconut cream, or full-fat coconut milk, or 1/2 cup cultured buttermilk and 1/4 cup mayonnaise.
- Add 1/2 teaspoon coconut vinegar, white wine vinegar, white balsamic vinegar, or soft tofu for flavor.
- Substitute for dill weed any other spice such as basil, marjoram, oregano, ginger, etc.
- Add 2 Tablespoons Parmesan, blue, or other cheese of your choice, stirred or blended in.

Soups and Stews

Every soup has its own story!
– Adam Nelson

Soup is my favorite thing to cook. My mother, Carlee, had a pot of some kind of soup on the stove all the time. She never used a recipe; she just had a basic idea for soup or chili and used what simple foods she had on hand. She stirred up a few ordinary ingredients for some memorable, delicious meals.

Soup can be as simple as putting your ingredients in a pot, covering them with water, and letting them simmer for a while. It is exactly that simple. You don't need fancy stock. The flavors of vegetables become delicious on their own when simmered together. Cooking is my Zen as I chop, stir, and create. Seasoning the pot creates layers of flavor as you adjust to taste, adding a dash of spice or a splash of vinegar.

Soup is a cook's playground. There are many types of soups, starting with broth and moving to chunky ones like chowders and stews, and to pureed and creamed ones like creamy tomato or butternut squash soup. When making soup, start with the end in mind. Picture the kind of soup you want to end up with and start from there.

Soups and stews taste even richer if made a day in advance. It seems like the flavors marry overnight and have children.

Vegetable Soup Recipe Template (makes about 11 cups)

Use what you have on hand and more or less of each ingredient. The amounts shown below are approximate suggestions. Use a large soup pot with a heavy bottom, or a Dutch oven.

Ingredients

5 cups washed, combined vegetables, greens, legumes, etc. Choose 2 or 3 aromatic vegetables like onions, carrots, celery, and garlic, and a combination of 2 or 3 other seasonal vegetables or legumes, and chop or dice them to make about 5 cups.

6 cups water, broth, or stock

Salt and spice to taste

Directions

1. Put vegetables in a large cooking pot.
2. Add enough water, stock, or broth to cover the vegetables, bring to a boil, cover, and simmer for 30 to 40 minutes or until tender, stirring occasionally.
3. Add more water if the liquid is cooking out.
4. Check the flavor at the end of the cooking time and adjust the seasoning if needed.
5. Leave as is or puree or mash for a creamy soup (see "How to Puree" below).

Other Possibilities

- Add beef chunks or browned hamburger for beef soup or stew.
- Use chicken stock, chicken, peas, diced carrots, and celery for chicken soup. Add noodles at the end of the cooking time and continue cooking until the noodles are done.
- Make it Mexican by adding chili powder, ground cumin, oregano; and fresh, chopped cilantro.
- Make it Italian by adding basil, marjoram, oregano, thyme, olive oil, and little meatballs.
- Make it Indian by adding curry powder, cumin, coriander, and ginger. Add bay leaf, cooked chickpeas, and cauliflower.
- Make it Moroccan by adding paprika, cinnamon, ginger, ground cumin, turmeric, and a dash of cayenne pepper. Add diced sweet potatoes, lentils, diced tomatoes, and lamb.

How to Puree

- Cook perhaps a little longer until all the ingredients are soft.
- Remove from the heat and mash with a potato masher. It won't be totally smooth but makes a nice thick soup.

OR:

- Use an electric emersion blender. It's fast and makes an amazing, creamy puree.

OR:

- Cool the soup and blend it in batches in a kitchen blender. Add half a slice of bread when blending for a smoother soup.

OR:

- Mash the soup through a strainer. It's messy, but it works if you don't have a blender.

Tips for Creamier, Thicker Soups

- Add about 1/4 cup cream, coconut milk, plain yogurt, or sour cream, and add more to taste if needed after it thickens.
- Remove a couple cups of soup from the pot, puree, and add back to the pot to thicken.
- Thicken with a roux: melt a few Tablespoons of your fat of choice in a pan and stir in the same amount of flour until it's a thick paste. Stir this light-colored paste into the soup, or continue stirring until it browns a bit before adding it. Dark brown roux is a flavor Cajun grandmas use in cooking.

- Kneed together equal parts butter or fat and flour to make a glob. Drop the ball into the soup and whisk to thicken.

- Whisk a Tablespoon or two of flour into a small bowl of water and stir in a little smaller amount of cornstarch, adding water as needed for a thin slurry. Drizzle this into the soup as you stir. Grain flours like white or wheat flour, chick pea, quinoa and others work.

- Grind nuts like cashews or almonds almost to a paste, then add to the soup. Soaking them beforehand adds to the creaminess.

Vegetables

I have made a lot of mistakes falling in love, and regretted most of them, but never the potatoes that went with them.
– Nora Ephron

Vegetables are the most versatile foods of all and aren't we always being told to eat more veggies? But how do you eat more vegetables if the same three vegetables you always buy are not on your Food Codes plan? Don't panic! Below are some really simple and easy ways to use a variety of vegetables in your cooking that you might come to love.

Some people don't like the texture, smell, or taste of certain vegetables. I wasn't fond of any vegetables except raw carrots and dill pickles when I was growing up – at my house vegetables were way overcooked. But many vegetables taste better after being cooked. How much heat, what kind of heat, and how long heat is applied while cooking are very important. Cooking vegetables makes them easier to eat. Our teeth and jaws can only take so much chewing! Vegetables become sweeter with cooking and it softens the tough cellulose fiber and boosts the release of certain nutrients. Cooking vegetables like tomatoes, carrots, spinach, kale, peppers, and cabbage provides more antioxidants than eating them raw. (I often include tomato in my lists and charts of vegetables, though it is actually a fruit.)

A few of the several ways to cook vegetables are to blanch, steam, stir-fry, bake, roast, boil, and grill. Adding fat, salt, and seasonings can make ordinary vegetables extraordinary. You can enjoy a simple baked potato or get your creative juices flowing and experiment with other methods of preparing vegetables.

You might need to eat some vegetables cooked and some vegetables raw, and by now you know how to determine this!

Vegetable Tips

- Soft vegetables like greens, tomatoes, zucchini, peas, and fresh beans need shorter cooking times.
- Hard vegetables like turnips, potatoes, carrots, and winter squash need longer cooking times and might need to be parboiled for some types of cooking like grilling.
- Size matters. When cooking vegetables together, cut pieces in the same sizes to cook evenly.
- Start with hard vegetables and add softer ones toward the end of the cooking time.

Roasted Vegetable Recipe Template (makes about 8 cups)

Roasting is simple and brings out the sweetness in even bitter vegetables. All the ingredients in this template can be varied. The measurements shown are approximate suggestions.

Ingredients

8 cups vegetables, washed and all cut into 1-inch pieces or all cut into 2-inch pieces

4 Tablespoons oil (prevents sticking, caramelizes for crispness and browning, and imparts flavor)

Salt, pepper and spices to taste

Directions

1. Preheat oven to 400 degrees.
2. Oil (or use vegetable spray) a shallow, flat pan, like a cookie sheet, or line the pan with parchment paper.
3. Combine cut vegetables, oil, and spices in a large bowl, and toss until well coated.
4. Spread vegetables in a single layer on the baking sheet. Don't crowd them together or they will steam rather than roasting. Give them space and roast in two pans if needed.
5. Roast 1-inch pieces for 30 to 35 minutes; 2-inch pieces for 40 to 45 minutes. Watch to make sure there is no burning. Stir about halfway through to expose all sides of veggies equally to the heat.
6. Roasting time varies. Poke with a fork to test for desired doneness. Don't worry if some of the veggies get dark on the edges; that adds flavor and crunch.

Tips

- To ensure equal doneness, roast soft vegetables separately from hard ones and combine after cooking to serve.
- Use high-temperature/low-smoke-point oil like olive oil, ghee (clarified butter), or grapeseed oil. Coconut oil and delicate oils burn more readily.
- Make a large batch of roasted vegetables, refrigerate, and use on salads, in wraps, as snacks, and add to cooked grains for a main dish.

Vegetable Combination Ideas

- Yellow (summer) squash, green beans, asparagus, tomatoes, garlic cloves, and mushrooms
- Rainbow: red and yellow bell peppers, zucchini, broccoli, and red onions
- Root vegetables: beets, potatoes, carrots, and parsnips
- Cruciferous vegetables: broccoli, cauliflower, and Brussels sprouts
- Butternut or acorn squash, red potatoes, and fennel
- Vegetable steaks (sliced 1 to 1 1/2 inch): cabbage, cauliflower, whole onion slices, and sliced sweet potato rounds

Other Possibilities

- No-oil method: Line pan with parchment paper. Toss vegetables in a large bowl with white or dark balsamic vinegar, lemon or lime juice, tamari, or liquid aminos; and spices.

- Bake vegetables in a covered baking dish for 15 to 20 minutes. Test with a fork for desired doneness.
- Steam vegetables over simmering water to retain flavor, tenderness, and nutrition. Flavor with sauce or eat plain.

Whole Cooked Vegetable Recipe Template

Forget all the chopping and slicing. Simply wash and trim a whole vegetable, then roast, bake, or slow cook. You might consider this a "vegetable roast."

Ingredients

1 whole vegetable such as a head of cauliflower, a cabbage, or a broccoli

4 Tablespoons butter, ghee, lard, coconut oil, or other flavorful oil (optional)

Minced or granulated garlic, salt, and pepper to taste

2 Tablespoons lemon juice, vinegar, or other acid (optional)

Directions

1. Wash vegetable and remove dirty or wilted outer layers. (No need to trim the green leaves from a cauliflower.) Pat dry.
2. Melt oil and mix in spices and acid of choice. Rub over vegetable.
3. Place in a slow cooker, cover, and cook on high for approximately 3 hours, then on low for approximately 5 hours or until a knife slides through the middle. (Cooking time varies depending on the denseness of the vegetable.)

4. Remove from slow cooker gently, place on serving plate, and drizzle the cooking juice over the top. Slice into wedges to serve.

Other Possibilities

- Add 2 cups diced ham, turkey, chicken, or other meat to the slow cooker before cooking and spoon on top.
- Dice a whole onion, shallot, red or green cabbage, broccoflower, or a mix of other vegetables like carrots and celery, add to the slow cooker before cooking, and spoon on top.
- Sprinkle with Parmesan or other cheese after cooking.
- Add a few medium-sized potatoes, small zucchini, or other whole veggies.

Vegetable Noodles and More!

Making noodles from fresh vegetables is so fun, and they're remarkably delicious! It can make a vegetable fan out of anyone. It's a creative way to eat your vegetables while enjoying grain-free "noodles." Simply cut a whole vegetable into strings of noodles by slicing spirally around the vegetable and eat them raw or lightly boiled. Use in soups, salads, and casseroles. Spiral-cut carrots and apples for salad. Zucchini noodles tossed with Asian dressing and other ingredients are tasty and healthy.

All you need is a spiralizer tool. You can get a hand-held spiralizer, which is easy to use, for about the price of this book. It's handier than a straight knife for softer veggies like zucchini, summer squash, cucumbers, and bell peppers, and also works great for carrots, parsnips, beets, and even onions. You can also get a large spiralizer that suctions to your counter and has a hand crank, which makes spiraling harder vegetables much easier.

Butternut squash noodles tossed with light oil, salt, and pepper and popped in the oven for a few minutes will be cleaned up at the dinner table. Zucchini, sweet potato, carrot, or parsnip noodles can be added to soup in the last few minutes of cooking.

But wait, there's more! Not only can you spiralize veggies and fruits, you can slice them into very thin sheets with a vegetable sheet-cutter. Potatoes, sweet potatoes, root vegetables, apples, zucchini, and many other vegetables and fruits can be sliced into sheets about as wide as your hand. One apple cut with a thin sheet-cutter makes a continuous sheet of apple that is about twelve feet long! I've heard this called a "real fruit roll-up."

Use vegetable sheets to replace flat pasta noodles for lasagna. Use them to replace tortillas for enchiladas and burritos or place chicken salad in them and roll them into wraps. Make your own crispy vegetable or fruit chips by cutting sheets into bite-sized pieces and baking them in the oven.

Preparing foods in a different way that changes the texture can make them more enjoyable. Get yourself and your family eating more whole vegetables and fruits in fun and delicious ways by noodling and sheet-cutting them.

Potatoes

My daughter Jennifer loves potatoes so much that when she was in high school, she would come home at midnight from a date and make herself mashed potatoes. That's true love!

Potatoes have supported nations as their main staple food. They can be boiled, baked, mashed, roasted, fried, scalloped, and more. Some types of potatoes might muscle-test for you better than others. Sweet potatoes often test as a good food. They come from a different plant family than other potatoes and vary from white to orange to red. They're sometimes called yams, but a yam is not a sweet potato. Yams grow up to five feet long; have a tough, bark-like skin; are fibrous and dry; and are native to Africa and Asia.

Baked Potato

Any kind of potato can be baked as below. When baking different kinds of potatoes together, make sure they are all close to the same size.

Directions

1. Preheat oven to 375 degrees.
2. Wash potatoes well and poke them several times with a fork to allow steam to release as they cook. If you don't do this you can end up with a potato grenade in your oven. (Ask me how I know!)
3. Coat them with oil and/or seasoning if you like, or just leave plain, and place on the oven rack or on a sheet pan or baking dish.
4. Bake for 45 minutes to an hour, depending on size. Test for doneness with a fork. When they're soft, they're done.
5. Sweet potatoes bake a little more quickly than other kinds.

Slow Cooker Potato: Cook for 8 to 10 hours.

Pressure Cooker Potato: Follow your pressure-cooker instructions; they can cook in 10 to 20 minutes, depending on size.

Baked Potato Bar

Combine baked potatoes with a salad bar for a healthy, hearty meal. Bake as many potatoes as needed, usually 1 per person, as above. I like to bake some russets and some sweet potatoes to be sure to cover everyone's food plan. Then put out several potato toppings using top foods from you and your family's Food Codes plans. Here are some possibilities:

- Avocado
- Any sliced, diced, shredded, chopped, grilled, or cooked vegetable such as broccoli, mushrooms, slivered cabbage, peas, etc.
- Crumbled or shredded cheese
- Sour cream or plain yogurt
- Any kind of sprouts
- Fermented foods like sauerkraut and kimchi
- Butter, coconut oil, olive oil, and other fats
- Chopped, shredded, ground, diced, or leftover meat, poultry, or seafood like crumpled bacon; cooked, diced chicken; ham; turkey; beef; or salmon
- Chili

Baked Winter Squash

Ingredients

1 medium squash, cut in half, such as butternut, spaghetti, or acorn
1 or 2 Tablespoons olive oil
Salt and pepper to taste

Directions

1. Preheat oven to 375 degrees.
2. Wash and dry squash.
3. Oil (or spray oil) a baking sheet or roasting pan with sides.
4. Be very careful when you cut the squash, as they are seriously tough. Slice off the stem end so it stands flat on your cutting board while slicing lengthwise.
5. Spoon out the seeds.
6. Brush the insides with the olive oil and sprinkle with salt and pepper if desired.
7. Place cut side down on the pan. (You can add water to cover the bottom of the pan to provide some steam if you prefer.)
8. Bake for about 40 minutes or until easily pierced with a fork. Large squash takes 10 to 15 minutes longer.
9. Remove from the oven and let sit for 10 to 15 minutes until cool enough to handle. Cut into portions and serve.

Other Possibilities

- Roast the squash whole. Pierce it several times before baking to release steam during cooking. Bake about an hour or until tender when poked with a fork. Remove from the oven and let cool for 15 minutes or until able to handle. Cut in half, pull out the seeds, and shred with a fork to serve.
- Use a pressure cooker, following the directions.
- Spaghetti squash is traditionally served with spaghetti sauce, and you can add meatballs if you like.
- Roast the seeds for snacks, just like pumpkin seeds.

Legumes

Three of the most beneficial, longevity promoting anti-cancer foods are green vegetables, beans, and onions.
– Joel Fuhrman

Beans, peas, lentils, and peanuts are all legumes. Peanuts are considered a nut, yet they grow underground and belong to the legume family. There are many species and varieties of legumes around the globe. They come in all shapes, sizes, and flavors from white to red, pink, spotted, and black. Also called pulses and dal, they're a worldwide food staple with many uses. They're inexpensive and very versatile, a good source of protein and fiber, and loaded with nutrients for overall health, yet are notorious for digestive issues such as gas and bloating. A compound in them called phytic acid can block some nutrients from being absorbed by your body. Read on to find out how to fix these problems.

Fast Pressure-Cooker Method to Cook Dry Beans

Don't shy away from cooking beans. This fast and easy method does not take all day.

Ingredients

2 cups dry beans (1 pound) (yields about 6 cups, equivalent to 3 1/2 to 4 16-oz. cans)

7 cups water

2 Tablespoons oil (to keep the liquid from foaming and clogging the air hole)

Directions

1. Pick through the beans, discarding any discolored or shriveled ones, and rinse and drain.

2. Combine ingredients in your pressure cooker. Never fill the pressure cooker more than half full.
3. Secure the pressure cooker lid and *cook according to your pressure cooker instructions*, about 22 to 25 minutes after cooker reaches pressure.
4. Dense beans like garbanzo beans (chickpeas) can take 35 to 40 minutes after cooker reaches pressure.

No-Gas Beans

The way a food is prepared affects its nutritional and "good for you" value. If beans have not muscle-tested as good for you, or have not been good *to* you in the past, preparing them in a different way might help you digest and assimilate them more happily.

Legumes are available dried or canned and ready to use. Soaking and sprouting dry legumes can make them more digestible and non-gas producing, and might be healthier than canned. Beans, peas, and lentils are threshed during harvest, but are not washed because the moisture would encourage sprouting. The outer coating of many beans contains sugars called oligosaccharides, which are hard for our stomachs to digest. They can cause gas when the intestines try to break them down. Soaking them removes field dirt, contaminants, and the indigestible starches which can cause gas.

Garbanzo beans are my favorite dry beans to cook from scratch. A fresh-cooked bowl of garbanzos with salt and pepper is simple to make and more delicious than you might expect. They have a rich, creamy texture and a nutty flavor that you just can't get from store-bought canned beans. I soak, sprout, cook, then freeze them in their cooking liquid in two-cup batches to use any time.

Other legumes include navy beans, great northern beans, kidney beans, pinto beans, black beans, lima beans, adzuki beans, cranberry beans, black-eyed peas, cannellini beans, and fava beans, to name a few. Legumes that don't need to be soaked include split peas and red, yellow, and brown lentils (green lentils are harder and benefit from soaking); these are usually dehulled before being packaged for sale.

Soaking Beans – Overnight Method

"Overnight" is not an exact measure of time; it just means from whenever you start the soak until the next day when you get around to cooking them. You can soak them for up to 24 hours if you drain them and change the water about half-way through.

Directions

For 1 pound (2 cups) of dry beans use 5 cups of water (yields about 6 cups, equivalent to 3 1/2 to 4 16-oz. cans). Double this for a larger batch.

1. Sort through the beans, discarding any dirt, rocks, or shriveled-up beans.
2. Rinse thoroughly with cool water.
3. Place beans in a bowl or cooking pan and cover with water.
4. Drain and rinse the next day and they are ready to cook.

Sprouting Beans

Directions

1. Follow the overnight soak method above, leaving the beans covered loosely – not sealed – to keep the moisture in.
2. Drain, rinse, and replace water once during the day and again before going to bed. Put them in the refrigerator overnight if it's very warm in your house.
3. Rinse the next morning and they're ready to cook. You can keep them covered in the fridge for a day or two. Large beans can be left to sprout for up to 3 days where it's less than 70 degrees. They need a good rinsing 2 or 3 times daily.

You may see small sprouts about coming out of the bean or bulging where the bean would sprout – where the bean has a "belly button." Small beans, like mung beans, and lentils grow a nice little sprout in 24 hours. Continue to sprout and rinse them for 2 or 3 days and eat them raw on salads or use them in a stir-fry. Black beans have a low germination rate and only a few might sprout. If your beans don't sprout they might be old and have gotten very dry. Soaking softens old beans, but they might not sprout and they might take longer to cook, though they're still okay to eat.

Stove-Top Beans Recipe Template

Ingredients

Soaked or sprouted beans from 1 pound of dried beans (yields about 6 cups, equivalent to 3 1/2 to 4 16-oz. cans)

Water – fill pot to 1 inch above the beans

Spices – aromatics like 1 or 2 bay leaves, 1/2 diced onion, 3 minced garlic cloves, or 1 teaspoon garlic granules

1/2 cup diced carrot (optional)

1/2 cup diced celery (optional)

2 or 3 teaspoons salt to taste

Directions

1. Place beans in a 4-quart Dutch oven or heavy-bottomed cooking pot, add water, spices, vegetables (if desired), and salt and stir.
2. Leave the lid off if you want firm beans for salads or toppings. Put the lid on, slightly askew, for creamy, soft beans for burritos, refried beans, and soups.
3. Bring them to a boil, then reduce to a simmer so the water is just lightly bubbling.
4. Start checking for doneness after 1 hour. They should take about 3 hours, but the time varies, and they get soft very quickly toward the end, so check more frequently toward the end. Dense beans like garbanzos take longer.
5. Check the flavor when done and season to taste.
6. Use immediately or cool and store for later use. Seal and refrigerate for 5 to 7 days; or freeze for up to 8 months.

Slow-Cooker Beans Recipe Template

Directions

1. Place all the ingredients in the "Stove-Top Beans Recipe Template" in a 5-quart slow cooker, again filling the cooker to 1 inch above the beans. Stir and cover.

2. Cook on low for 6 to 8 hours. Test for desired firmness from time to time, as the time can vary.
3. Season, cool, and store as above.

Pressure-Cooker Beans Recipe Template

Ingredients

Use the same ingredients as in "Stove-Top Beans Recipe Template," adding 1 Tablespoon of oil to keep the liquid from foaming and clogging the air hole.

Directions

1. Place all ingredients in a 6- or 8-quart pressure cooker. Never fill the pressure cooker more than half full.
2. Secure the pressure cooker lid and *cook according to your pressure cooker instructions,* about 12 to 18 minutes after cooker reaches pressure.
3. Dense beans like garbanzo beans can take 20 to 25 minutes after cooker reaches pressure.

Tips for Legumes

- Salting both the soaking water and the cooking water aids in moisture retention, enhances flavor, and keeps the beans from breaking apart.
- Split peas and red, yellow, and brown lentils have been hulled and may be rinsed, then cooked (green beans are tougher and benefit from soaking). Soaking or sprouting is not needed and they cook quickly, so check them often to ensure they don't get mushy.
- Black beans and black-eyed peas are soft beans and cook much faster than other beans.

> *You might be a redneck if you consider pork and beans to be a gourmet food!*
> *– Jeff Foxworthy*

Hummus Recipe Template

Hummus is a nutritious dip or spread for vegetables, chips, or crackers; a sandwich spread on bread or flatbread; a spread for lettuce rolls and salad wraps; and can be used in salad dressings or as a sauce for grains. *Hummus* is the Arabic word for chickpea and *garbanzo* is the Spanish word for chickpea, but you can use any kind of legume in this recipe. Use a food processor for a creamy consistency. A blender makes it even creamier, but you'll need more liquid so it will be thinner.

Ingredients

4 cups home-cooked legumes (or 2 15-oz. cans, drained and rinsed)

1/3 cup liquid (Combine water or liquid from the cans, olive oil, and lemon juice. Make a little extra in case you need it.)

Spices to taste (optional)

Directions

1. Add legumes to a food processor (or blender) and give them a quick pulse.
2. Add the liquid to the processor and process until smooth. The longer it mixes the lighter and creamier the hummus. Add liquid if needed to make it thinner.
3. Taste and mix in spices in small doses.

Tips

- Try it with white beans, black beans, split peas, yellow or red lentils, or frozen edamame. All make delicious and different hummus flavors.
- Spoon into a serving bowl and eat plain or with a drizzle of fragrant olive oil and/or a sprinkle of more spices or fresh, chopped herbs.
- It will keep in the refrigerator for a week.

Other Possibilities

- There are no rules for flavoring hummus; just play with what your taste buds like, adding flavors and spices when processing. Try fresh garlic, cumin, paprika, smoked paprika, sundried tomatoes, green or black olives, toasted pine nuts or walnuts, or anchovy paste.
- For more traditional hummus, mix in 1/4 to 1/2 cup sesame tahini paste while processing.
- Use a different oil that you like or that tests best for you.

Grains, Seeds, and Nuts

"Eat more whole foods and grains," is resounding in health headlines. I will show you not only how to easily get whole grains into your diet, but how to get more out of them nutritionally. And if these foods have not been the best for you in the past, they might be now using the easy and fast preparation methods below. You can actually change the *energy* of these wonderful foods!

Various grains and "seed grains" can replace wheat and rice if those foods are not your bests. They cook up much the same as rice and you can even cook them in a rice cooker or pressure cooker.

Soaking and roasting improve the digestibility of grains and seeds, remove molds and other toxins, and might increase their nutritional value. Soaking starts the germination process, which multiplies and activates nutrients like vitamins A, B, and C.

Due to legislation in the US regarding safe food handling, most of the "raw" nuts we buy are not truly raw. Shelled nuts may have been steamed or dried with heat to kill pathogens and reduce moisture that encourages growth of molds and bacteria. Nuts can be a healing food, full of beneficial nutrients and good fats. Most nuts won't sprout, but soaking makes them easier to chew and good for snacking.

The soaking method is the same for grains, seeds, and nuts as for legumes, though the time needed varies. Some will sprout, and some won't. Some don't benefit much from soaking. You can muscle-test to see if soaking or roasting is beneficial for you. Simply ask if it would benefit you to soak or sprout them. Soaked grains, seeds, and nuts can be kept in the refrigerator for several days, after which they must be frozen or dried, as they can grow mold and bacteria.

Toasting turns up the flavor, sterilizes, and enhances digestibility. Toast before boiling for use in recipes.

Toasted Grains, Nuts, and Seeds

1. On the stove: Toast in a dry skillet over medium heat for 3 to 5 minutes, stirring to prevent scorching, until they're just slightly brown and have a fragrant smell.

2. In the oven: Preheat oven to 350 degrees. Spread on a rimmed baking sheet and toast for 10 to 15 minutes. This takes more time but reduces the risk of scorching, which makes them bitter.

Cooking Grains and Seeds

I used to shy away from making rice because I could never get it right, not even in a rice cooker. The only time I had good rice was when eating out! If you are confused like I was about whether to buy long grain, short grain, wild, or brown rice, or the myriad of other kinds of rice and grains and how in the world to cook them, read on. (I'll just call them all grains from here forward for simplicity.)

I love having grains on hand as a basic ingredient for a bowl-based meal or to add to salads, wraps, and stir-frys. Grains can be the base ingredient for any meal. They can be cooked in large batches and refrigerated or frozen in serving amounts for quick, easy meals at any time. Warm them up with a little water or broth or toss with veggies and dressing for a salad. Use them as a base for a one-dish meal in a bowl, in wraps, or add to canned soup for extra goodness.

Cooking grains is literally as simple as boiling water. With a little experience you will learn to recognize the different stages of doneness by observing changes in color, texture, and taste. You will shy away from buying those expensive processed boxed meals.

You can cook all types of grains exactly as you would cook pasta. You don't need to remember a dozen water-to-grain ratios. All you need is a large pot of boiling water. The extra water lets them shed starch, which is what leads to a gummy pot of rice when using conventional ratios.

Grains cook more quickly if soaked for a few hours before cooking.

Watch the grain as it cooks and keep in mind the average cooking times in the chart below. Grains that cook quickly, like millet and amaranth, need to be watched closely so they don't turn mushy.

Cooking Times for Grains and Seeds

Cooking Times	Types of Grains and Seeds
No cooking	bulgur wheat: pour 1 1/2 cups boiling water over 1 cup bulgur and let it stand for 30 minutes. Drain off excess water and use
10 to 20 minutes	amaranth, couscous, buckwheat, millet
20 to 25 minutes	cracked wheat, kasha, quinoa, steel cut oats, white rice
40 to 60 minutes	pearl barley, brown rice, freekeh, wild rice, sorghum, whole oats
65 to 80 minutes	kamut, farro, rye, spelt, triticale, wheat

Yields

1 cup dry grain yields about 3 cups cooked.

1 cup dry buckwheat or millet yields about 4 cups cooked.

1 serving of cooked grain is 1/2 to 1 cup, depending on the meal.

Grain and Seed Recipe Template

Surprisingly simple! Don't worry about measuring if you're cooking a batch to freeze or keep in the fridge for random meals; just eyeball the grain and know that it is going to make about 3 times the dry amount when cooked.

Ingredients

Grain or seeds of choice

Water

Salt

Aromatic veggies to add flavor such as bay leaves, garlic cloves, a quartered onion or shallot, celery stalk, citrus peel, etc. (optional)

Directions

1. Fill a large cooking pot 1/2 to 3/4 full with water, and salt well. (Add some salt and taste the water – it should taste salty.) Bring to a full boil over high heat. Add veggies if desired and return to a boil.

2. Add grain gradually to pot while stirring to keep from clumping. Keep water at a steady boil. Lower the heat a little if it threatens to boil over.

3. Set a timer for about 10 minutes *before* the grain should be done cooking according to the "Cooking Times" chart above.

4. Check for doneness and stir every couple of minutes until done the way you like it, whether still firm or soft.

5. Strain through a fine strainer (removing veggies first if you used them) and serve.

Tips

- To keep grain from getting gummy while you prepare the rest of your meal, place two paper towels under the pan lid and replace the lid so that the paper towels stay up under the lid. They will absorb the moisture rising from the grain.
- Grains absorb salt and other flavors when used in recipes, and can leave a dish tasting bland and boring. Keep in mind the five essential flavors – the salt, acid, fat, sweet, and spices you will be using in your recipe, and season and taste while preparing it and again before serving, especially for salads and grain dishes that you've made in advance.
- Adding aromatics and spices to the cooking water, or using broth instead of water, adds flavor.

Pilaf Recipe Template (serves 4 to 6)

Ingredients

2 to 3 Tablespoons oil, butter, ghee, light olive oil, or another fat

1/2 to 1 cup chopped vegetables – bell pepper, onion, celery, broccoli, kale, peas, slivered or diced carrot, sliced mushrooms – whatever you like

4 cups cooked grain – any grain or combination of grains. Grain cooked in chicken or vegetable broth is especially good for pilaf.

Salt, fresh ground pepper, and seasonings such as minced garlic, basil, rosemary

1/2 to 1 cup roasted pine nuts, walnuts, or other nuts (optional)

Directions

1. Add fat and vegetables to a large skillet or pot and sauté over medium heat until tender. Add hard vegetables first and soft vegetables when the hard ones soften a bit.
2. Add the grains, nuts, and seasonings, and stir until warmed.
3. Serve in a warmed serving dish.

Tips

- Traditional pilaf is mostly rice or quinoa, with diced onion, carrot, and celery. Shake it up by mixing grains and adding colorful vegetables and tasty spices.
- Leftover rice pilaf makes good stir-fried rice.
- Make a cold salad with leftover pilaf by stirring in vinaigrette dressing, cucumber chunks, and fresh tomatoes.

Stir-Fry Recipe Template (serves 4)

Ingredients

3 to 5 cups cooked grain

2 or more Tablespoons oil or broth such as sesame oil, olive oil, grapeseed oil, vegetable broth, bone broth

2 to 3 cups chopped vegetables such as squash, onion, broccoli, pea pods, carrot, cauliflower, bell pepper, green beans, celery

1/4 cup sauce such as coconut aminos, coconut milk, tamari, peanut, or nut

1 to 2 cups cooked protein such as chicken, turkey, beef, pork (optional)

1 to 3 Tablespoons aromatic vegetables and spices such as garlic, ginger, cilantro, shallots, grated lemon peel, dried or fresh chilies

Directions

1. Warm up a pan or skillet over low heat with a little oil in the bottom, and add the cooked grain. Toss and stir every few minutes so it doesn't burn, or keep it warm in a 200 degree oven while doing the next steps.
2. Add oil or broth to a large skillet over medium-high heat. If using garlic and ginger, add those now. Add firm veggies first and cook for about 5 minutes. Add soft veggies when hard ones soften a bit, and cook for 2 to 3 minutes.
3. Add a thin sauce now, toss, and simmer for a couple of minutes. (Add thick sauces like peanut or nut just before serving.)
4. Stir in cooked protein until warmed.
5. Add aromatic vegetables or spices (and thick sauce if using that).
6. Serve over the warm cooked grain.
7. Garnish with fresh herbs like cilantro, a squeeze of lemon or lime juice, or chopped nuts.

Casserole Recipe Template (serves 6 to 8 people)

Ingredients

2 to 3 cups cooked grain

2 cups sliced vegetables such as zucchini, yellow squash, Brussels sprouts, onion, celery, cauliflower, mushrooms

1 to 2 cups cooked protein such as chicken, turkey, ground burger of any kind, tuna, seafood, black or red beans (optional)

1 to 1 1/2 cups sauce such as spaghetti sauce, creamed soup, bone broth gravy, yogurt, sour cream, diced tomatoes, coconut milk

Salt, pepper, and spices

1/2 to 1 cup toppings such as bread crumbs or cubes, shredded cheese, bacon crumbles, toasted nuts, crumbled whole grain chips, water chestnuts, olives, fresh herbs

Directions

1. Preheat oven to 350 degrees.
2. Lightly oil a 9"x13" baking dish.
3. ***Method 1***

    Combine and mix all ingredients in a mixing bowl. Spread mixture into the baking dish and sprinkle with topping.

    Method 2

    Spread the grain across the bottom, add vegetables a layer at a time, then a layer of the protein. Spread or drizzle sauce on top and sprinkle with toppings.
4. Bake 40 to 60 minutes, until top is brown and bubbly.

Nut, Grain, and Seed Milk Recipe Template (makes 1 quart)

Homemade non-dairy milk tastes nothing like the watered down or unnaturally sweet versions from the grocery store. And you know what's in it when you make it! A label on a non-dairy milk can list more than a dozen ingredients, some questionable.

Ingredients

1 cup raw, unsalted nuts (almonds, Brazil nuts, hazelnuts, pistachios, walnuts, pecans, cashews, macadamias); raw, unsalted seeds (pumpkin, sunflower, sesame, hemp, chia, flax); or cooked grain

4 cups water

Pinch of sea salt, vanilla, or sweetener (optional)

Directions

Soak

1. Soak these: almonds, Brazil nuts, hazelnuts, pistachios, walnuts, pumpkin seeds, sunflower seeds, sesame seeds. No need to soak: cashews, macadamia nuts, hemp seeds, chia seeds, flax seeds, cooked grain.
2. Place in a bowl and fill with distilled water to 2 inches above the nuts/grains/seeds. Let sit overnight or up to 24 hours in a cool place. Longer soaking gives the milk a smoother texture.
3. Drain and discard soaking water. No need to remove almond skins.

Blend

1. Combine nuts/grains/seeds with 4 cups of water and salt in a blender. Secure the lid well, start the blender on low speed, and increase it to high speed for about 2 minutes or until well blended.
2. Add another 1 to 2 cups of water if you want a thinner milk, and blend.
3. For flavor add a pinch of salt, a couple drops of vanilla, or a pinch of sweetener if desired, and blend.

Serve

- Use unstrained over oatmeal, granola, or muesli; in smoothies; or in seed puddings like chia pudding.
- To use strained as a beverage, strain over a bowl through a fine mesh sieve lined with cheese cloth, a thin cotton towel, or a nut milk bag. Press and squeeze out the liquid from the pulp. Discard the pulp.
- Transfer to an airtight container and refrigerate. Shake before using.

Freeze

- Make and freeze extra batches to save time and cleanup. Homemade milks don't have the preservatives that store-bought milks do, so they won't keep as long in the refrigerator. Pour the milk into freezer-safe containers and freeze. Thaw in the refrigerator, and shake well or blend when thawed.
- Freeze in ice cube trays and pop a couple of cubes into a smoothie!

Other Possibilities

- For chocolate milk, add 1/3 cup cocoa powder and sweetener of your choice.
- For berry milk, add freeze-dried raspberries or blueberries.
- Use herbal tea instead of water.

Bread

No yoga exercise, no meditation in a chapel filled with music will rid you of your blues better than the humble task of making your own bread.
– M. F. K. Fisher

My dad was a baker, and he made the best bread and pastries I have eaten anywhere in the world. When I asked my son Matt, who has followed his own passion as a chef, what his favorite thing to cook is, his countenance relaxed and he sighed, "Bread. Sourdough bread." He said that he found a peaceful pleasure in kneading and making bread by himself in the kitchen.

Sourdough bread muscle-tests good for many people, even those who have not been able to eat wheat products. This could be due to the wonderful fermentation process of the sourdough culture, which seems to make the grain more digestible. The yeast used in regular bread bothers some people.

If you have never made bread, it's really very easy to make. You can use sourdough or another type of grain or a combination of grains. Please refer to TheFoodCodes.com for my sourdough bread recipe.

Muscle-test to find out what grains and seeds are best for you. You can find readymade breads made with those that you can eat. Make sure that sourdough bread has been made with real sourdough starter.

Garbanzo Flour Socca Bread

This is a no-grain bread using garbanzo bean flour. It makes a delightfully mild-tasting flatbread. Even a beginning cook can make it, and it's a great substitute if wheat bread is not good for you right now.

Ingredients

1 part garbanzo bean flour (chickpea flour)

1 part water

2 to 3 Tablespoons oil

Salt to taste

Example: 1 cup garbanzo bean flour and 1 cup water make a 10-inch pan, or four servings.

Directions

1. Whisk together garbanzo bean flour and water until completely smooth. Let rest for at least 20 minutes to let them meld. (You can rest it for several hours.)
2. Preheat oven to 450 degrees.
3. Oil an oven-proof pan or skillet and place it in the oven.
4. When the oven is preheated, carefully remove the pan with an oven mitt and pour the batter into the pan, tilting to coat the bottom completely. Return to the oven.
5. Cook for 15 minutes until golden and slightly crisp. (Place under broiler briefly to brown and crisp the edges if you like, watching carefully to be sure it doesn't burn.)
6. Remove from the oven, drizzle with a little oil, serve like flatbread, and eat it hot. Top with a flavorful oil or seasonings if you like.

Tips

- Make pancakes by simply spooning the batter onto a greased griddle. Serve as you would any pancake.
- Make crepes by spooning the batter into a hot greased skillet and swirling the pan to thin and spread the batter. Serve as a savory or sweet crepe.
- Use pancakes or crepes like tortillas for tacos or tortilla rolls.

- Use as a pizza crust. (See Adam's Socca Bread Pizza in the "Cooking with The Food Codes" chapter.)
- Make a pizza, taco, or sandwich bar for a family gathering
    - Make several small pancakes, crepes, or pizza crust rounds.
    - Put out a choice of toppings such as sliced or shredded raw or cooked vegetables, olives, meats, poultry, and fish.
    - Put out a choice of sauces such as tomato sauce, pesto, and alfredo sauce.
    - Provide choices with all five essential flavors for variety.

Meat, Poultry, Fish, Seafood, and Eggs

Chopped vegetables *release* their flavors in recipes because we normally chop them into pieces to prepare them, exposing more surfaces. Chopping poultry, seafood, and meat into small pieces causes these proteins to *absorb* flavor. So to enhance the flavor of proteins, cut them into pieces before cooking to soak up seasonings and get that tasty caramelizing effect of browning. Pounding a chicken breast flat and seasoning it makes it tastier than a big baked chicken breast. Stir-fry is tasty because the meat is chunked small and absorbs the flavorful sauce.

Leaving the bone in (and the skin on in the case of poultry and fish) provides extra nutrition and flavor when cooking meat, poultry, and seafood. Pressure cooking is a good way to roast whole meats and poultry.

Tips for Quick Meals

- Cook a turkey or chicken, cut into portion sizes, and freeze to use later.
- Bake a tray of chicken breasts, thighs, and legs and freeze or refrigerate individually so you can pull out one or several depending on how many you're cooking for.
- Cook a quantity of ground meat or poultry, divide into portion sizes, and freeze or refrigerate to use later.
- Cook a whole fish such as wild-caught salmon, cut into portion sizes, and freeze or refrigerate to use later.

Other Tips

- Save bones, fat, skin, and trimmings from meats, poultry, and fish to make bone broth.
- Save leftovers for soups, stews, and wraps.

Frittata Recipe Template (serves 4)

Frittatas are great for brunch, a quick dinner, or weekend guests, and they will be impressed! You can double the ingredient quantities and bake them in a 9"x12" baking dish.

Ingredients

6 to 8 whole eggs

1 cup or more cooked vegetables such as onion, bell pepper, spinach, carrot, tomato, mushrooms

1/2 cup cooked protein such as bacon, sausage, ham, poultry, fish, seafood

Spices and/or herbs, fresh or dried, such as basil, paprika, smoked paprika, garlic, rosemary, thyme, cilantro, parsley (use half as much dried as fresh)

1/2 cup topping like shredded cheese, sour cream, yogurt, sliced green onions (optional)

Directions

1. Preheat oven to 350 degrees
2. Oil an 8"x8" baking pan or an 8- to 10-inch cast iron skillet.
3. Whisk together eggs in a large mixing bowl.
4. Stir in the vegetables, protein, and seasonings.
5. Pour the egg mixture into the baking pan.
6. Bake for 30 to 45 minutes until eggs are firm, not runny.
7. Add topping and serve.

Tips

- Use leftovers for the vegetables and/or proteins and add a grain if you have leftover grain.
- Make a chunky mirepoix and substitute it for the vegetables. (See the next section for the mirepoix recipe.)
- Makes great leftovers and it's even good cold.

Sauces

When you're feeling "saucy," take a couple hours and whip up some homemade batches of sauce to have on hand. Freeze or refrigerate them to use whenever you need them. Making your own sauce is a breeze, and homemade sauce has flavor goodness and nutrition that you won't find in any jarred sauce.

Almost every savory soup, casserole, grain dish, and roast starts with common vegetables. When chopped very small these vegetables disappear into the sauce.

As always, don't worry about exact ratios in the following recipes. Choosing aromatic ingredients for sauces is part of the creative cooking process. Sometimes you will use a certain ingredient and sometimes you won't, even when cooking the same dish, depending on what you have on hand and what tests good for you at the time.

Mirepoix

As mentioned above in "Aromatic Foods," cooks worldwide have used mirepoix for centuries to add flavor to their cooking, regardless of what it's called in different languages. Onions, carrots, and celery are probably in your fridge right now. Substituting one or two ingredients magically changes the flavor to Spanish, Oriental, Eastern, and other cuisines.

Make mirepoix as a foundation for almost any cooked dish, then add the other ingredients and finish the recipe. It's just that simple. For example, you can scatter it in the bottom of a roasting pan for mouthwatering roasted meats, fish, or vegetables. Use it as a go-to foundation for soups, stews, casseroles, and stir-frys.

Ingredients (makes enough to flavor a 6-to-8-serving recipe)

2 parts onion, diced (example 1 cup)

1 part carrot, diced (example 1/2 cup)

1 part celery, diced (example 1/2 cup)

2 Tablespoons butter or fat

Salt and pepper to taste

Directions

1. Dice vegetables all the same size. Small pieces cook faster and almost melt into a sauce. Large pieces keep their form and add substance to soups and stews.
2. Stir vegetables and fat in a heavy-bottomed skillet or soup pot over medium-high heat. Cook for a few minutes, then turn the heat down to keep the sauce from burning and continue cooking until tender. Add salt and pepper.

Tips

- To use in stock or a pot of boiling grain or beans, don't worry about dicing. Just halve the onion, leaving the skin on, chop the carrot and celery into 2 or 3 chunks, and add whole sprigs of fresh herbs. Fish out the chunks or drain the sauce through a strainer before adding other ingredients.
- Add mirepoix's raw ingredients to stock or broth for a lighter flavor.
- For sweeter mirepoix to use in a white sauce or light gravy, replace carrots with leeks, parsnips, or mushrooms.
- Broth can be substituted for the fat, but fat is much better at releasing the flavors.
- Prepare a large quantity of diced vegetables and freeze them in portion sizes, either together or individually, OR freeze whole vegetables on trays, put them into large freezer bags, and take out the amount you need each time you make mirepoix. Blanching (see "Basic Cooking Methods" above) the vegetables first makes a better product, but you can freeze them without blanching. They will be a little mushy when thawed, but you can add them to the pan frozen and still have a nice sauce.

Mirepoix Variations

Variation	Main ingredients	Fat	Flavoring additions	Serve with or use as flavor base for:
Italian/ Spanish	2 parts onion 1 part carrot 1 part celery	olive oil	garlic, bay leaf, parsley, basil, pancetta or prosciutto, balsamic vinegar	pasta, orzo, grain, veggies, soup, poultry, meat, fish, omelets, frittatas, pizza
Marinara Sauce	2 parts crushed or chopped tomato 1 part onion 1 part garlic/ shallot combined	olive oil	sweetener, basil, thyme, oregano	pasta, orzo, grain, veggies, soup, poultry, meat, fish, omelets, frittatas, pizza, dipping sauce
Cajun/ Creole	2 parts onion 1 part celery 1 part green bell pepper	olive oil or butter	garlic, paprika, tomato or tomato paste, Cajun seasoning, andouille sausage	rice, orzo, grain, veggies, soup, poultry, meat, fish, omelets, frittatas

Variation	Main ingredients	Fat	Flavoring additions	Serve with or use as flavor base for:
Chinese	1 part onion 1 part green onion 1 part garlic, ginger (combined or to taste) 1 part combined red, green, and yellow peppers	light, flavored olive oil, grapeseed oil, or sesame oil	cilantro; whole, dried, red chilies; Chinese 5 spice; hoisin sauce; hot chili sauce; oyster sauce; rice vinegar; sweetener	soba noodles, pasta, grain, veggies, soup, poultry, seafood, meat, fish, omelets, frittatas
Indian	2 parts crushed or chopped tomatoes 1 part onion 1 part garlic/shallots combined	ghee (clarified butter)	tomato, eggplant, curry, cumin, cardamom, fenugreek, turmeric, coconut milk	grain, beans, lentils, garbanzos, veggies, soup, poultry, lamb, goat

Variation	Main ingredients	Fat	Flavoring additions	Serve with or use as flavor base for:
Thai (curry)	1 part onion 1 part green onion 1 part garlic, chilies (combined or to taste) 1 part combined red, green, and yellow peppers	oil or coconut milk	peanut butter or nut butter, green onion, cumin, coriander, fresh basil lemongrass, shrimp paste, fish sauce, lime juice and zest	grain, veggies, soup, shrimp, chicken, eggs, frittata, wrap sandwiches

CHAPTER 14

Cooking with the Food Codes

Using the Food Codes for Simple, Quick Meals

If you cook extra quantities and plan ahead, your grab-and-go meals are in your fridge. You can throw a meal together if you have greens, prepped or cooked vegies, grains, proteins, and readymade or bottled sauces.

A "bowl" is any foods you combine together in a bowl or dish for a complete meal. Look online for ideas to get creative. You can make any kind of bowl from a smoothie breakfast bowl to savory and unlimited combinations. Use the chart below for ideas and refer to each of the food sections above for ideas.

Meal-Planning

1. Choose the type of meal you want.
2. Choose the main food base, fresh or precooked.
3. Choose one or more other fillings, fresh or precooked.
4. Choose one or more toppings, fresh or precooked.
5. Choose the flavor – sauce and spices.

Step-by-Step Meal-Planning Chart

1	2	3	4	5
Meal type	Main food base	Fillings	Toppings	Flavor: sauces and spices
Salad	green salad, wedge salad, salad bar, melon salad	grain, beans, meat, poultry, seafood, eggs, avocado	sprouts; sesame, pumpkin, sunflower, or flax seeds; nuts; olives; capers; dried fruit; cheese; sourdough croutons	vinaigrette, tahini, hummus, purchased dressings
Bowl	grain; beans; fresh, spiralized vegetables like zucchini or yellow squash; cooked spaghetti squash	meat, poultry, seafood, eggs	chopped nuts, sour cream	vinaigrette, mirepoix, tamari, tahini, homemade or bottled salsa, any flavor in the "Mirepoix Variations" chart above

1	2	3	4	5
Meal type	**Main food base**	**Fillings**	**Toppings**	**Flavor: sauces and spices**
Wrap made with lettuce leaves, collard leaves, nori, tortillas OR sandwich made with socca, sourdough, rolls, etc.	greens, fresh or cooked vegetables	grain, beans, meat, poultry, seafood, eggs	cheese, grapes, olives	hummus, pesto, mayonnaise, mustard, any flavor in the "Mirepoix Variations" chart above
Sauté or Stir-Fry	grain, beans	fresh vegetables of choice; fresh, spiralized zucchini or yellow squash noodles	sesame seeds	tahini, tamari, any flavor in the "Mirepoix Variations" chart above

Food Codes Sample Recipes

Below are examples of real Food Codes plans used to make dishes and recipes. You might even find that some of these recipes work with your lists.

Rachel

Rachel is a mom of five busy kids, and she works from home. She has learned to muscle-test foods and cook for her family using the Food Codes method. She can put together a few ingredients in a slow cooker after she gets the kids off to school in the morning and have dinner waiting in the evening.

Rachel's Food Codes List

	Rachel's High-Energy Foods	**Rachel's Low-Energy Foods**
Vegetables/ Legumes	bok choy; broccoli; cabbage; carrot; celery; cucumber; bibb and iceberg lettuce; spinach; kale; tomato; onion; sweet pepper; red and white potato; sweet potato; beet; black beans; chickpeas; portabella, shiitake and button mushrooms; butternut squash; zucchini; white beans; lentils	asparagus, Brussels sprouts, corn, eggplant, green beans, kale, hot pepper, ginger, peas, radish, turnip, soy beans
Fat/Oil	beef fat tallow, butter, ghee, chicken fat, olive, pork lard	hemp, margarine, peanut, soy, vegetable

Cooking with the Food Codes

	Rachel's High-Energy Foods	**Rachel's Low-Energy Foods**
Meat	beef, chicken, duck, elk, goose, lamb, turkey, venison	liver, pork, ham, bacon, rabbit
Fish	cod, halibut, mackerel, salmon, tilapia, tuna	catfish, flounder, swordfish – no shellfish
Grain	amaranth, barley, millet, oats, quinoa, basmati rice, brown rice, wild rice	wheat, corn, white rice, rye, spelt
Herbs/Spices	basil, bay, celery seed, chive, cilantro, cumin, garlic, mustard seed, oregano, parsley	chili pepper, clove, dill, fennel, ginger, mint
Salt	most salt very good	white table salt
Dairy/Non-Dairy	kefir, sour cream, coconut milk, natural cheddar cheese	milk, soy milk, soy products, most cheese
Nuts/Seeds	almond, cashew, coconut, macadamia, hazelnut, walnut	hemp, sunflower, pecan, peanut

Rachel's Easy Vegetable Soup (makes about 11 cups)

Ingredients

Mirepoix: 1 diced onion, 2 diced carrots, 4 sliced celery stalks with leaves, 4 minced garlic cloves

3 Tablespoons coconut oil

5 cups or more combined vegetables: chopped green cabbage, zucchini, unpeeled red potatoes

1 medium to large sweet potato, unpeeled, cut into 1- to 2-inch pieces

2 bay leaves

1 teaspoon dry basil

1/2 cup chopped parsley or 2 Tablespoons parsley flakes

Water to cover vegetables

Kosher salt to taste

Directions

1. Sauté onion, carrots, celery, and garlic together with the coconut oil in a large cooking pot until tender.
2. Add the vegetables and spices.
3. Add enough water to cover the vegetables and bring to a boil.
4. Reduce heat, cover, and simmer for 30 minutes or until tender, stirring occasionally.
5. Add more water if liquid is cooking out or for more broth.
6. Check flavor at the end of cooking time and add more seasoning if wanted.

Cooking with the Food Codes

Options

- Vegetable beef soup: by adding beef, stew meat, or hamburger with beef broth in place of water
- Chicken noodle soup: by adding chicken, chicken broth, and noodles
- Serve with crusty sourdough bread and a tossed green salad, seasonal fruit salad, or melon salad.

Rachel's Black & White Bean Chicken Chili (makes about 8 servings)

Rachel loves chili, but chili peppers, mild or hot, are not a good food for her. She says that she loves the flavor but not the heat. Note that neither chili pepper nor paprika spices are in her food list; sweet peppers are best for her.

Ingredients

4 cups cooked black beans (or 2 15-oz. cans)

4 cups cooked white beans (or 2 15-oz. cans)

2 onions, diced

2 sweet red peppers, diced (or 8-oz. jar)

3 to 6 garlic cloves, minced (or 1 to 3 teaspoons garlic granules)

2 15-oz. cans diced tomatoes (or 1/2 to 2 cups packed, diced, fresh tomatoes)

3 cups cooked chicken (or meat from 1 cooked chicken)

1 teaspoon dried oregano

2 teaspoons ground cumin

Sea salt to taste

Directions

1. Drain and rinse the black beans. Do not drain the white beans; include their juice in the chili.
2. Put all ingredients in a slow cooker and stir.
3. Slow cook for 6 to 8 hours.
4. Serve with sour cream and shredded natural cheddar cheese.

Options

- Substitute any kind of beans, green peppers, or ground meat.
- Add 2 cups chicken broth for a soup-like chili.
- Make it vegetarian by omitting the chicken.
- Serve with non-corn chips like quinoa or rice chips, mild salsa, and small dishes of chopped onion, cilantro, and guacamole. Make it a fiesta!

Cheryl, Adam, and Avery

Cheryl and Adam are young parents of a three-year-old daughter, Avery. Whoever gets home from work first starts dinner. They have learned to plan and shop on the weekend for their coming week's meals. Avery can be a picky eater. She "accidentally" drops food from her plate that she doesn't like, to be snatched up by Berkley, the family's black lab.

Cheryl's Food Codes List

	Cheryl's High-Energy Foods	Cheryl's Low-Energy Foods
Vegetables/ Legumes	asparagus, Brussels sprouts, bok choy, broccoli, cabbage, celery, cucumber, eggplant, lettuce, spinach, kale, tomato, onion, sweet and hot pepper, red potato, radish, sweet potato, beet, black beans, chickpeas, button mushrooms, butternut squash, spaghetti squash, zucchini, lentils	carrot, corn, white and red potato, turnip, soy beans
Fruit	avocado, lemon, watermelon, orange, papaya, pineapple	banana, red and green grapes
Fat/Oil	beef fat tallow, butter, ghee, grapeseed, chicken fat, almond, olive, pork lard	hemp, margarine, peanut, soy, vegetable
Meat	beef, chicken, elk, bacon, turkey, rabbit, venison	
Fish	bass, cod, halibut, salmon, tilapia, trout, tuna, whitefish	catfish, flounder, swordfish – no shellfish

	Cheryl's High-Energy Foods	**Cheryl's Low-Energy Foods**
Grain	amaranth, buckwheat, millet, oats, quinoa, brown rice, wild rice	wheat, corn, white rice, rye, spelt
Herbs/Spices	basil, celery seed, chili, chive, cilantro, cumin, garlic, mustard seed, oregano, parsley, rosemary	mint
Salt	Celtic salt, Redmond salt, Himalayan pink salt	white table salt
Dairy/Non-Dairy	kefir, yogurt, coconut milk, natural cheddar cheese, goat cheese	milk, soy milk, soy products, most cheese
Nuts/Seeds	almond, coconut, macadamia, hazelnut, walnut; chia, flax, and sunflower seeds	hemp, peanut
Sweeteners	coconut sugar, date sugar, honey, maple syrup, molasses	artificial sweeteners, stevia, xylitol
Other	eggs	

Cheryl's Brussels Sprouts (serves 4 to 6)

Cheryl wows family and friends when she cooks this side dish.

Ingredients

1 pound (about 4 cups) Brussels sprouts, sliced in half

1/2 pound bacon, chopped into 1-inch pieces

2 cups mushrooms, sliced or cut in halves

4 to 6 garlic cloves, sliced

Salt and pepper to taste

1/2 cup Parmesan cheese for topping

Directions

1. Rinse Brussels sprouts, remove any wilted leaves, trim off the ends, and cut in half. Steam or parboil until barely tender. Dry on paper towel.

2. Steam or drop into salted boiling water for about 8 minutes or until fork tender.

3. Fry the bacon in a large skillet until crisp. Drain on a paper towel, reserving the bacon fat in the skillet.

4. Add the mushrooms and garlic to the bacon fat and sauté until tender and slightly browned. Toss bacon and Brussels sprouts into the skillet.

5. Season with salt and pepper, remove from heat, place in a serving dish, and top with Parmesan cheese.

Cheryl's Pressure-Cooker Spaghetti Squash

Adam and Avery love this spaghetti-like cooked squash. Adam likes it with butter and a drizzle of honey, and Cheryl loves it savory with salt and pepper. Avery likes the texture, which is fun to slurp up like spaghetti noodles.

Spaghetti Squash is a sweet, mild-tasting, watery squash. The fibers hold together in spaghetti-like strands when stripped out with a fork. It can be cooked to an al dente, crunchy texture or a very soft texture. Both ways are delicious.

Use your pressure cooker's directions for cooking. If you don't have a pressure cooker you can easily bake this recipe instead. (See the "Baked Winter Squash" recipe above.)

Ingredients

1 spaghetti squash

Salt and pepper to taste

Directions

1. Rinse spaghetti squash off or wipe with clean, damp cloth.
2. Be very careful when slicing the squash as it's very tough! Slice off the stem end, very carefully slice in half lengthwise, and spoon out the seeds.
3. Put in a pressure cooker with 1 cup water.
4. Cook for 12 minutes from the time the pressure cooker is up to pressure (or follow your cooker's instructions).
5. Scrape out spaghetti-like insides with a fork, add salt and pepper, and serve in one of the optional ways below.

Options

- Toss with coconut oil to accent the already sweet taste of the squash.
- Sprinkle with brown sugar and a dollop of butter.
- Serve with spaghetti sauce. Kids love the spaghetti-like texture.
- Serve cold in salads.

Avery has been raised to eat "real" healthy food. Cheryl nursed her for a good beginning and made her baby foods from fresh vegetables and fruits. Though Avery sees other kids eating sweet kiddie treats and wants to eat those too, using the Food Codes method helped her parents know what foods are best for her and how to give her better choices that she will eat. Many foods are "good" to "neutral" for Avery; note her high-energy foods and low-energy foods in the chart below.

Cheryl found a boxed macaroni and cheese product that doesn't contain a lot of additives and tests good for Avery, which they prepare for her when rushed for a quick meal. Instead of juice or soda pop, a drink that delights Avery is sparkling mineral water. She also loves to sip mild herbal tea from a pretty teacup.

The Food Codes: Intuitive Eating for Every Body

Avery's Food Codes List

	Avery's High-Energy Foods	**Avery's Low-Energy Foods**
Vegetables	beet, carrot, cabbage, celery, cucumber, kale, lettuce, onion, sweet pepper, spinach, most squash, pumpkin, red potato, sweet potato, tomato, most beans and lentils	corn, white potato, soy beans
Fruit	avocado, blueberry, fig, lemon, strawberry, watermelon, papaya	
Fat/Oil	avocado, beef fat tallow, butter, ghee, almond	margarine, peanut, soy, vegetable
Meat	chicken, elk, turkey, venison	lamb
Fish	salmon, trout, tuna, whitefish	
Grain	buckwheat, millet, oats, quinoa, organic wheat pasta, quinoa pasta	corn
Bread/Flour	sourdough, garbanzo, buckwheat	
Herbs/Spices	basil, garlic, parsley	
Salt	Himalayan pink salt	white sea salt, table salt

	Avery's High-Energy Foods	**Avery's Low-Energy Foods**
Dairy/Non-Dairy	whole milk, buttermilk, yogurt, coconut milk, hard natural cheese	soy milk, soy products
Nuts	almond, coconut, walnut	
Sweeteners	date sugar, honey, maple syrup	artificial sweeteners
Other	eggs, almond butter, dried figs, raisins, dried apricots, dried goji berries, chamomile tea, mild herbal tea, natural mineral water	soda pop, cranberry juice, apple juice, peanuts, peanut butter

Avery's Favorite Buckwheat Pancakes

A nearby breakfast café where Avery's family likes to treat themselves to breakfast on weekends serves buckwheat pancakes. Avery loves them at home now, too. Top them with a natural sweetener like real maple syrup, a drizzle of honey, nut butter with natural jam or yogurt, or a sprinkle of date sugar.

Ingredients

1 cup buckwheat flour

1 teaspoon baking powder

1/4 teaspoon baking soda

1/4 teaspoon salt

1 1/4 cups buttermilk

1 beaten egg

1 Tablespoon honey

1/4 teaspoon vanilla (if desired)

1. In a bowl, stir together buckwheat flour, baking powder, baking soda, and salt.
2. In another bowl whisk together buttermilk, egg, honey, and vanilla.
3. Gradually combine the flour mixture with the buttermilk mixture, then mix well and let sit for about 10 minutes while heating a skillet or griddle over medium heat.
4. Spoon batter onto greased, hot skillet or griddle. When the middles of the pancakes are full of bubbles and the edges are slightly dry, flip them. Cook another 1 or 2 minutes until lightly browned.

Tips and Options

- For lighter pancakes let the batter sit 15 minutes so more moisture is absorbed by the buckwheat flour.
- Add 1 teaspoon cinnamon.
- Instead of buttermilk use 1 1/4 cups milk or non-dairy milk combined with 1 Tablespoon lemon juice or 1 Tablespoon vinegar. This thickens and acidifies the milk.
- For blueberry pancakes, drop several blueberries on top of pancakes while they're on the griddle before turning.

Avery's Real Fruit Snacks

You can use freeze-dried fruits in this recipe if you prefer. It's fast and easy to make a batch and package them into small bags.

Ingredients

Dried figs, diced or sliced into small pieces

Dried apricots, apples, pears, and/or ginger, diced or sliced into small pieces

Dried blueberries, raspberries, strawberries, or cranberries

Raisins, currants, goji berries, or other dried fruits

Walnut chunks, cashew nut pieces, or other easy-to-chew nuts (almonds, for example, don't work well because they're hard for children to chew)

Granola or granola bits

Directions

Toss together any amount or combination of fruits, nuts, and granola. Seal in an airtight container or put into individual serving bags.

Keep in the refrigerator or freezer for several months for freshness.

Other Possibilities

- Add freeze-dried ingredients like peas, tomato chunks, carrots, and bell peppers.
- Add small crackers and/or pretzels.

Adam was eating out every day for lunch and grabbing fast food. He gained weight, felt sluggish and cranky, and started having liver pain and a very unhappy digestive system. He used his Food Codes to create a cleanse and dropped twenty-five pounds in the first two weeks.

Adam said, "This cleanse has given me depth into just how unhealthy I was actually eating. I am feeling way better replacing bread and fries with quinoa and vegetables. I love quinoa. I never thought I would say that!"

Adam's Food Codes List

	Adam's High-Energy Foods	Adam's Low-Energy Foods
Vegetables/ Legumes	asparagus, Brussels sprouts, broccoli, cabbage, cauliflower, celery, cucumber, lettuce, kale, tomato, onion, sweet and hot pepper, red potato, radish, sweet potato, spinach, beet, carrot, black beans, chickpeas, button mushrooms, butternut squash, yellow squash, zucchini, lentils	soy beans, corn, jicama, mushrooms
Fruit	apple, avocado, cranberries, huckleberries, strawberries, lemon, lime, orange, papaya, pineapple, fig	
Fat/Oil	almond, avocado, butter, ghee, flax, grapeseed, olive, beef tallow,	corn, peanut, vegetable, soy bean
Meat/Poultry	beef, elk, bacon, bison, turkey, rabbit, venison	
Fish	bass, cod, lobster, scallop, salmon, tilapia, trout, whitefish	
Grain	amaranth, millet, quinoa, brown rice, wild rice	corn, wheat, white rice

	Adam's High-Energy Foods	**Adam's Low-Energy Foods**
Bread/Flour	sourdough, garbanzo	all wheat, rye, rice, corn, soy
Herbs/Spices	basil, celery seed, chili, chive, cilantro, cumin, dill, garlic, mustard seed, oregano, parsley, rosemary, thyme, turmeric	
Salt	Celtic sea salt, Himalayan pink salt, Redmond salt	table salt, white sea salt
Dairy/Non-Dairy	kefir, coconut milk, Irish cheese	cow's milk, ice cream, soy milk, soy cheese
Nuts	almond, coconut, hazelnut, macadamia, walnut	peanut
Sweeteners	date sugar, honey, maple syrup, molasses	all artificial sweeteners, rice syrup, white sugar, xylitol
Other	eggs, dark chocolate	tofu

Adam's Socca Bread Pizza

Pizza is Adam's favorite food, and he loves how good and satisfying socca bread is, so he uses what they have on hand to make his socca bread pizza, like grilled veggies; leftover burger, sausage, bacon, or chicken; readymade pizza sauce; and sometimes specialty cheeses. His favorite is using leftover grilled veggies as the main topping.

Dough Ingredients

1 cup garbanzo bean (chickpea) flour

1 cup water

2 to 3 Tablespoons olive oil

Sauce Ingredients (no cooking!)

1 or 2 cloves fresh garlic

1/4 to 1/2 onion, coarsely chopped

1 14 oz. can diced or crushed tomatoes (approximately 1 3/4 cups)

1 teaspoon honey

1 teaspoon basil

1/2 teaspoon Himalayan pink

sea salt fresh ground

pepper to taste

Directions

1. Whisk together flour and water until completely smooth. Let rest for at least 20 minutes for flour to absorb water.
2. Preheat oven to 450 degrees
3. Oil an oven-proof pizza pan, a 9"x12" baking pan, or a large oven-proof skillet and place it in the oven.
4. When the oven is ready, carefully remove the pan and pour in the batter, tilting to coat the bottom. Return to the oven.
5. Cook for about 15 minutes or until the edges are set. Remove from the oven but keep the oven hot.
6. Prepare the sauce:
    a. Pulse whole garlic cloves in food processor to dice.
    b. Add chopped onion and pulse 2 or 3 times to break up.

c. Add tomatoes. (Drain the tomatoes if you want a thicker sauce.)

d. Add honey and spices.

e. Process, scraping down sides until smooth.

7. Spread the sauce on the crust and add toppings and any additional seasonings you like. Refrigerate extra sauce for up to 5 days or freeze for up to 3 months.

8. Return to the oven until bubbly or cooked, about 10 minutes.

9. Cut and serve.

Adam's Marinara Sauce (makes about 2 cups)

Adam's marinara sauce is based on the mirepoix recipe template in the "Recipes" section under "Sauces." Use as a chunky pizza sauce or as a savory dip for toasty socca bread slices. Delicious tossed with pasta or grains. Use warm or cold.

Ingredients

1 Tablespoon olive oil

1/2 to 1 finely chopped onion (up to a cup if you like onion)

1 14 oz. can diced or crushed tomatoes (approximately 1 3/4 cups)

1 teaspoon natural sugar

1 teaspoon basil

1/2 teaspoon Italian seasoning

1/2 teaspoon sea salt or to taste

Directions

1. Add oil to a medium sized, heavy-bottomed skillet and heat over medium heat for 1 minute.

2. Add onions and sauté until tender.
3. Add tomatoes, sugar, and spices and bring to a simmer, stirring often for 10 to 15 minutes. Taste and adjust spice.

Other Possibilities

- Use fresh, firm tomatoes (with either sauce recipe), about 2 1/2 cups, chopped.
- Add fresh spices like cilantro, parsley, chopped chilies, or garlic.
- Use any spices to your taste, and chili pepper for extra heat.

Tips

- Refrigerate extra sauce for up to five days.
- Freeze sauce in amounts for pizza topping using a muffin tin. When frozen, pop out the pucks and store in a freezer-proof container. They will keep for about three months.

Kathleen

Kathleen is an author, speaker, and marketing strategist now in her sixties. A couple of years ago she found herself standing in front of the mirror, "butt naked" as she says, and was not happy with the view. She knew what she needed to do in the area of exercise and training to get back into shape and she jumped into a training program. She changed her diet drastically, omitting her bad foods.

She says, "The result was nothing short of miraculous." Today she's sixty pounds lighter. "The first time someone called me slim I literally looked around to see who they were talking about. Oh my gosh! It's me!"

Kathleen has won numerous racing medals since her decision to get healthy and is now training for a triathlon.

She thanks the Food Codes for her food program. "I'm loving the way I'm feeling and know the special food protocol specific to my needs is a huge factor!"

Kathleen's Food Codes List

	Kathleen's High-Energy Foods	**Kathleen's Low-Energy Foods**
Vegetables/ Legumes	artichoke, asparagus, avocado, beet, Brussels sprouts, broccoli, cabbage, celery, collards, cucumber, leek, lettuce, spinach, kale, tomato, onion, sweet pepper, red potato, sweet potato, spinach, black beans, chickpeas, butternut squash, yellow squash, zucchini, lentils, green olives	hot peppers, soy beans, corn, jicama, mushrooms
Fruit	apple, avocado, blueberries, strawberries, fig, lemon, watermelon, orange, papaya	bananas, all grapes, grapefruit
Fat/Oil	avocado, butter, coconut, ghee, flax, grapeseed, olive, walnut	corn, peanut, lard, palm, vegetable, soy bean,
Meat/Poultry	lamb, turkey, chicken	pork
Fish	salmon, tuna	all shellfish

	Kathleen's High-Energy Foods	**Kathleen's Low-Energy Foods**
Grain/Seeds	millet, oats, quinoa, wild rice, chia seed, flax seed, hemp hearts	corn, wheat, white rice, hemp,
Bread/Flour	sourdough, garbanzo	all wheat, rye, rice, corn, soy
Herbs/Spices	basil, celery seed, cilantro, cumin, curry, dill, garlic, mustard seed, oregano, parsley, rosemary, turmeric	chilies
Salt	Himalayan pink salt	table salt, white sea salt
Dairy/Non-Dairy	yogurt, goat yogurt, coconut milk	most dairy, rice milk, soy milk, tofu, soy cheese
Nuts	almond, coconut, macadamia, walnut	peanut
Sweeteners	date sugar, honey	all artificial sweeteners, brown sugar, white sugar, xylitol
Other	eggs, dark chocolate	tofu, milk chocolate, sugar free chocolate, popcorn, rice cakes, egg protein, pea protein, rice protein, soy protein, coffee

Kathleen's Power-Packed Wake-Up Drink

This will start your day off perfectly. Kathleen enjoys this drink every day; it's perfect before a good workout or run.

Ingredients

Green tea

1 Tablespoon organic flax seeds

1 Tablespoon organic chia seeds

1 Tablespoon organic hemp hearts (optional)

1 Tablespoon medium-chain triglyceride (MCT) oil

1 medium-sized apple, chopped into small pieces

1 lemon, peeled

Directions

1. Brew a cup of green tea, letting it steep for 20 minutes.
2. Put all ingredients in a blender and blend at high speed for one minute or until very smooth.
3. Drink immediately, but slowly.

Kathleen's Power-Packed High-Protein Breakfast Bowl

Perfect *after* that run or workout!

Ingredients

2 organic eggs

1 teaspoon coconut oil

1/4 cup high-quality cooked wild rice, heated

1/2 small to medium avocado, cut in bite-sized pieces

Directions

1. Cook eggs sunny side up in oil.
2. Mix together eggs, rice, and avocado.

Kathleen's Homemade Turkey Soup

Ingredients

4 to 5 quarts water, depending on size of turkey carcass

1 turkey carcass

6 small red potatoes, cut into pieces

3 stalks celery

1 large onion, cut into pieces

1 to 2 teaspoons pink Himalayan salt

1/4 teaspoon ground pepper

1 cup fresh chopped parsley

1 cup fresh chopped cilantro

4 large carrots, diced (optional)

Directions

Phase I

1. Boil the water
2. Add the turkey carcass
3. Reduce the heat to simmer
4. Cover and simmer for one hour

Phase II

1. Use a fine mesh strainer to drain the broth into a clean soup pot.
2. Remove the remaining turkey meat from the carcass.
3. Chop the turkey that came off the carcass into small pieces.

Phase III

1. Add the chopped turkey to the strained broth.
2. Bring to a boil and add the rest of the ingredients.
3. Reduce heat and simmer until the vegetables are tender, approximately one more hour.

APPENDIX 1

Measurement Conversion Chart

US Dry Volume Measurements	
MEASURE	**EQUIVALENT**
1/16 teaspoon	dash
1/8 teaspoon	pinch
3 teaspoons	1 Tablespoon
1/8 cup	2 Tablespoons (= 1 standard coffee scoop)
1/4 cup	4 Tablespoons
1/3 cup	5 Tablespoons plus 1 teaspoon
1/2 cup	8 Tablespoons
3/4 cup	12 Tablespoons
1 cup	16 Tablespoons
1 pound	16 ounces
US liquid volume measurements	
8 fluid ounces	1 cup
1 pint	2 cups (= 16 fluid ounces)
1 quart	2 pints (= 4 cups)
1 gallon	4 quarts (= 16 cups)

US to Metric Conversions	
1/5 teaspoon	1 ml (ml stands for milliliter, one thousandth of a liter)
1 teaspoon	5 ml
1 Tablespoon	15 ml
1 fluid ounce	30 ml
1/5 cup	50 ml
1 cup	240 ml
2 cups (1 pint)	470 ml
4 cups (1 quart)	.95 liter
4 quarts (1 gal.)	3.8 liters
1 oz.	28 grams
1 pound	454 grams

APPENDIX 2

Measurement Conversions for Pans and Dishes

Inches	Centimeters
9-by-13-inch baking dish	22-by-33-centimeter baking dish
8-by-8-inch baking dish	20-by-20-centimeter baking dish
9-by-5-inch loaf pan (8 cups in capacity)	23-by-12-centimeter loaf pan (2 liters in capacity)

APPENDIX 3

Oven Temperature Conversions

Fahrenheit	Celsius
275º F	140º C
300º F	150º C
325º F	165º C
350º F	180º C
375º F	190º C
400º F	200º C
425º F	220º C
450º F	230º C
475º F	240º C

ABOUT THE AUTHOR

Lana Nelson, an internationally renowned food intuitive, has helped people from six continents overcome personal health obstacles through making food choices unique to their needs.

Lana uses the power of energy techniques from her own health challenges for healing, muscle-testing, and intuition to help her clients. She discovered that a major solution to healing was as close as her kitchen cabinets and refrigerator.

Lana is a licensed massage therapist and a reiki master teacher who counsels in nutritional, herbal, homeopathic therapies and quantum biofeedback technology. She is also a seasoned practitioner of Dr. Bradley Nelson's The Emotion Code and The Body Code. She lives with her family in a beautiful setting in Montana.

ACKNOWLEDGMENTS

I acknowledge Dr. Bradley Nelson, creator of the Emotion Code and the Body Code, and his wife, Jean, for their wonderful examples of helping the world be a better place.

To Kathleen Gage: high fives! Kathleen is a rock star business coach and author who shoots out the gate with a bang to get to the finish line. She taught me and showed me by example how to get to the finish line with this book. She was there to uplift, advise, and cheer me on when I was winded and to carry me with one foot dragging when I couldn't go another step further.

A really big hug to my patient, witty, generous, and very intuitive publisher, Lynne Klippel. Thank you for your excellent professional advice and teaching me so much about writing. Thanks, too, for saving my readers from all the excessive details that were edited from the book! Her team at Thomas Noble Books, Gwen Hoffnagle and Sarah Barrie, made this book beautiful and easy to read.

Thanks to Melanie Boroczyk, my wonderful website creator, who has an eye for design and color. She not only makes things pretty, she is very savvy about making technology work well.

To my great mastermind buddies: thank you for all your support and business wisdom and yummy dining when we get together. Alli Berman, Lynn Jordan, Lynn Taylor, Kimberley Marooney, and Karolyn Bloom, you are inspiring women.

I also acknowledge my mom and dad, Carlee and Jerry Rasmussen, who among many other things helped me have a wonderful relationship with food. Good homemade food was at the core of all our family gatherings. Jerry was a baker and made the best bread and pastries in the world. I have never had better.

Big hugs to my sisters, Judy and Terri, and brothers, J. Clair, Kent, and Harold, who all survived my early cooking attempts! They have always been there for me, along with their wonderful spouses. And I also send an apology to my dear siblings — please forgive me for locking you in the basement to force you to eat that horrible batch of oatmeal cookies I made when I was eleven. I didn't know any other way to get rid of them.

I acknowledge the Creator of all for my most blessed and happy life and for creating such interesting, delightful food.

GET MORE FROM LANA

Lana does personal consultations via phone for people who want individual instruction on using the Food Codes to create glowing good health.

For more information on her work, recipes, and other helpful information, visit TheFoodCodes.com

Be sure to download your free copies of the Food Codes Food List at TheFoodCodes.com/lists.

Did you like this book?

Today's readers depend on reader reviews to help them find useful books. If you liked this book, please do me a big favor and leave an honest review at Amazon.com, even if you purchased the book elsewhere. Your opinions matter and are very much appreciated!

Made in the USA
Coppell, TX
17 October 2021